DANCE-MOVEMENT THERAPY: MIRROR OF OUR SELVES
The Psychoanalytic Approach

Elaine V. Siegel, Ph.D., A.D.T.R.
Private Practice
Huntington Sta., N.Y.

Institute for Psychotherapeutic Studies
Babylon, N.Y.
Antioch University
Keene, N.H.

Copyright© 1984 by Human Sciences Press
Published by Human Sciences Press, Inc.
72 Fifth Avenue, New York, New York 10011

Printed in the United States of America
123456789

Library of Congress Cataloging in Publication Data

Siegel, Elaine V.
  Dance-movement therapy.

  Bibliography: p.
  Includes index.
  1. Dance therapy. 2. Movement therapy.
3. Psychoanalysis. I. Title. &DNLM: 1. Dance
therapy. WM 450.5.D2 S571dé
  RC489.D3S54 1984   616.89'1655   83-22639
  ISBN 0-89885-157-2
  ISBN 0-89885-193-9 (pbk.)

DEDICATION

For Eugene J. Siegel without whose staunch
emotional support this book would never have been
written, and in memoriam, for Melanie.

CONTENTS

ACKNOWLEDGEMENTS

Editors and Publishers of the following journals and publications have kindly given permission to include portions of the papers previously published:

AAHPERD for Focus on Dance VII
American Journal of Dance Therapy
American Academy of Psychotherapy for Voices:
   The Art and Science of Psychotherapy
Human Sciences Press
Journal of the American Psychoanalytic Association
International Universities Press

My appreciation and thanks go to Bette Blau, Michele Rose, Patti Schmitt and Linda Salz-Citron, all registered dance therapists, for their unflagging professional support and the contribution of examples using psychoanalytic interpretation in dance-movement therapy.

All interpretations from the German are the writer's own.

FOREWORD

Elaine V. Siegel is a psychoanalytically trained pioneer in the use of movement therapy. She correctly asserts that "most psychic phenomena have their residue in our bodies to be used and translated" and describes the ways and means of bringing the physical state of being into a patient's awareness so that the stress may be reduced. This knowledge than becomes a springboard for the examination of the individual's psychic economy as a whole. Her aim: to re-create a homeostasis between psyche and soma and thereby promote integration.

This volume addresses itself to a treatment modality—movement therapy—that has only recently become recognized as a subspecialty among the many approaches for the alleviation of emotional disorders that have arisen since the late 1940s. Some behavioral scientists have long been aware of the usefulness of this treatment tool as an adjunct therapy, but others have declared an unwarranted rejection of a proper study of this modality because of its roots in dance and esthetic experience. Dr. Siegel not only addresses herself to these issues with dedication, but formulates and structures a body of clinical observations and theoretical conclusions. Through her lens the reader can trace the evolution of a therapy and of a therapist who has striven valiantly and succeeded in creating a scientific basis for movement therapy.

Her conceptualizations along psychoanalytic lines have rendered a service to dance-movement therapy and all creative arts therapy. To her, motility is part of the ego apparatus, imprinted on the psyche out of life's experiences and influenced through the mediation of the ego. Thus motility may be considered in a sense an "ego function" as it were and can be studied more fully than heretofore. In this connection it should be noted that few psychoanalysts, with some notable exceptions, e.g., Mittelman, Spitz, Kris, Levine, Kestenberg have conducted as intensive motility pattern observational studies on either children or adults as has the author.

Dr. Siegel has exhaustively researched the psychoanalytic literature and has found corroboration for many of her theoretical propositions in the work of the major theoreticians of psychoanalysis. She finds Freud's early formulations most applicable to her therapeutic vision, and her dissatisfaction with some present translations led her personally to retranslate from the German relevant portions of Freud's work as they pertained to motility. In strengthening the theoretical underpinnings of dance-movement therapy through the careful application of psychoanalytic principles, she enriches the creative arts therapies, makes practitioners in these fields further aware of the responsiblilty engendered by practicing such therapies, and provides guidelines for those creative-arts therapists who wish to add psychoanalytic depth to their work.

Dr. Siegel's case histories are straightforward, accurately observed accounts. They lean heavily on her perception of a psychoanalytic developmental psychology. That her approach "works" becomes apparent not only in the way her patients respond and grow, but also in the fact that she has been able successfully to transmit for over a decade her particular synthesis of psychoanalytic thought and dance-movement therapy to students and supervisees. This definitive work extends psychoanalytic thought into a new area and will not soon be superceded.

Charles W. Socarides, M.D.
Clinical Professor of Psychiatry
Albert Einstein College of Medicine
New York City

PREFACE

When I lecture and teach about the kind of dance-movement therapy I have developed, people often respond to what I have to say by asking: "Where can I read about this?" There are many psychoanalytic works I could recommend. But with the notable exception of Bernstein's (1979) Eight Theoretical Approaches to Dance-Movement therapy there aren't even any attempts at complete conceptualizations of the largely nonverbal phenomenon known as dance-movement therapy in print. Dance-movement therapy in general is a new treatment tool. A comparative study is not yet possible. The innovative work that is now taking place in studios, clinics, hospitals, and research laboratories has not yet reached publication. Case histories and explorations of the various properties of human motor behavior now available attest to the value of dance expressions within life's vicissitudes and contribute to the understanding of motility, but together they do not provide a consistent theoretical framework that can be the basis for specific hypothesis and predictability in treatment. In this book I hope to have laid the groundwork for such a theoretical structure.

It is not a job I undertook lightly. I am aware of the pitfalls and incompleteness inherent in such work. I hope that others will add and expand where my vision failed.

I cast about for years in the search for a synthesis and a synthesist that would help me to explain and investigate what I was doing as a dance-movement therapist. Egopsychoanalytic and developmental theory offered the springboard from which I developed "Psychoanalytic Dance-Movement Therapy."

I soon realized that this title meant different things to different people. This book will help to clarify what I mean. My work with clients and in-depth involvement with psychoanalysis and dance-movement therapy as a student, analysand, and clinician showed me that I was on a course of discovery not many others had followed. Inevitably, I saw that my work rested on two pillars: dance and psychoanalysis. What I was doing was the synthesis of the two.

Out of this synthesis grew a fledgling theory. Statements about how I built this theory comprise the contents of this book. In my theory building I cincluded some aspects of psychoanalytic thought and excluded others. It was a painful intellectual struggle at times because I was faced with the necessity of negating or disagreeing with some aspects of Freudian metapsychology and theory. I also had to make a decision as to which psychoanalytic thinkers would be included in depth, which not.

My choice fell upon those theoreticians who could provide basic principles consistent with both Freud's and my own thinking: i.e., I excluded thinkers who were either building their own theories based upon different assumptions than my own or whose work was derivative of other than Freudian theories. Thus, I did not include Alexander Lowen and other Bioenergeticists because their backgrounds are Reichian. I did not include Sweigard's Ideokinesis, Alexander Technique, Feldenkrais' Awareness through Movement or Rolfing, because in these modalities inner happenings are accepted without investigation or linkage to life experience. Because these therapies provide no consistent techniques for the dissolution of resistances or transferences they cannot be called psychoanalytic. Freud (1914) says specifically: "It may thus be said that the theory of psychoanalysis is an attempt to account for two striking and unexpected facts of observation. . . the facts of transference and resistance. Any line of investigation which recognizes these two facts and takes them as a starting point of its work has a right to call itself psychoanalysis. . . ''(pg. 16)

The work of Dr. Judith Kestenberg, despite the fact that she is a psychoanalyst, also did not fit into my conceptualizations. Kestenberg views motor behavior as an area suitable for diagnosis and primary prevention, not therapy. She believes that even if her primary prevention may help to re-educate mothers' movement patterns in relation to their children, this does not necessarily prevent trouble from occuring in other developmental phases. In other words,

Kestenberg does not view motility as a suitable agent for therapy but advocates its use for re-education. Yet in reading some of Kestenberg's case material and the way she talks about movement, it is easy to understand why some dance-movement therapists think of her as a psychoanalyst who is sympathetic to psychoanalytic dance-movement therapy. Kestenberg observes movement from a psychoanalytic point of view but does not use movement psychoanalytically. When it comes to the use of movement she culls techniques from Laban and others to produce desired educational effects. She also specifically embraces the classic psychoanalytic postion that movement and interpretation should not be intermingled. (1967, 1971, 1975, 1977). But the kind of dance-movement therapy I do rests heavily on precisely the combined use of movement and psychoanalytic interpretation as I reiterate throughout this book.

The influences that shaped my vision are manifold. I must assign equal weight to Freudian thought and methodology and to dance in the evolution of my therapy and treatment modes. Classic ballet and Haitian primitive dance molded my own behavior in tandem with both orthodox and ego psychoanalytic thinking. Most prominent as guides and teachers in my journey toward "something new" were Liljan Espenak, D.T.R., Dr. Robert C. Lane, Dr. Geraldine Pederson-Krag, Rubin Blanck, M.S.W., and Dr. Colin Greer. They provided the structure which allowed me to bring some order and hope to those who asked for it.

INTRODUCTION

Why is our Body, for us, the mirror of our being,
unless it is a NATURAL SELF?

M. Merleau-Ponty

I

Dance-Movement Therapy, as of this writing, stands in the professional world among the therapies as a very young, healthy adult,
ready to conquer with skill, enthusiasm, and strength many areas
that other therapies have eschewed. It is not uncommon today to find
dance-movement therapists in mental hospitals, clinics, and special
schools who can enter the universe of this autistic child and that
schizophrenic adult with compassion and insight. But, after the contact has been made, what happens? Is there a predictable course of
treatment events? What is it the dance-movement therapist con-
tributes beyond the immediate event of having made contact? There
are those who argue that it is enough in itself to facilitate body contact
with the touch-me-not aspects of the autistic client, or to loosen the
rigidity of catatonia in a circle dance. No doubt this is true on some
level. But all too often the touch-me-not child returns to his or her environment still untouchable by any but the dance-movement
therapist and the catatonic resumes a retreat behind incontrovertible
walls just as often when a particular "dance lady" is not available.

Does dance-movement therapy, then, commit the same folly as
many a brilliant young adult in the first glow of autonomy? Does it
promise what it cannot deliver? Or is there some health-giving magic
in —what? The process of creating a dance? In the fact that client and
therapist engage in the same activity at once? In moving itself? One
could speculate in this vein forever and come up with part answers
that fit individual situations. What is needed instead is a coherent
structure that allows for the formulation of predictions in treatment
that can be validated by the client's subsequent behavior.

1

INTERPRETATION IN
DANCE-MOVEMENT THERAPY

The work presented here is written from the point of reference of such a theory: namely, psychoanalytic ego psychology which includes motility as an ego apparatus and verbal interpretation. Thus, it differs from the conceptualizations of other dance-movement therapists. Rather than dealing with the phenomenon of movement and its properties exclusively, verbalizations, clarification (Rogers, 1951; Bibring, 1954) and psychoanalytic interpretation (Loewenstein, 1951; Kris, 1951; 1956) are seen as a form of intervention as important as the movement sequences.

This is not typical of the field. But it is commitment to psychoanalytic interpretation along with movement that makes it possible for clients to develop their strengths. Interpretation does not mean talking about what either therapist or client are doing, nor is it appropriate to introduce issues not raised by the client either verbally or nonverbally. All interventions need to be based on something the client has produced. Depending on the client's needs one might spend a good deal of time preparing for interpretation first. That is, the therapist might clarify, explain, or confront until the time for a properly constructed psychoanalytic interpretation arrives. This interpretation then would aim at resistance and defense before id material, at transference, and at the inclusion of genetic propositions (Loewenstein, 1956). The emphasis might rest on the dynamic interplay between inner forces which produces a specific effect in the mental life of the client, or it may deal specifically with the influences of the past upon the present.

There is currently no evidence in the literature that indicates the use of psychoanalytic interpretation within dance-movement therapy in just this manner.

To the observer it could seem that helping patients become aware of how they behave is considered more important in dance-movement therapy than helping them to see why they behave as they do (Geller, 1978). Yet Marian Chace, the great originator of dance therapy, already knew that feeling something was not enough in and of itself. When working with children who have special problems she observed that "those who have been helped are the ones who know what happened" (undated biographical note, Chaiklin, 1975, p. 11).

This knowing what happened is a component in any therapy that fosters change. It would be difficult to meet a client who has changed permanently without knowing what happened. Those who merely feel good and don't know why, disappear from sessions after a while and return to conflicted forms of behavior at the next time of stress in their lives. Quite simply, one needs to understand on many levels, including the cognitive one, what has happened.

Movement is an aspect of human experience that bears the imprint of past life but is subject to influence in the present. But by focusing primarily on movement in its expressive aspects, dance-movement therapists unwittingly propagate the splits that verbal therapies also foster. By ignoring or downplaying the intellectual and cognitive functions of their clients, they shift the emphasis from one aspect of human behavior to another. Thus, the split between body and mind frequently remains, to the detriment of the client's further evolution.

This mode of doing therapy was encouraged by primary therapists who were comfortable with the idea that moving about in dancelike fashion might be recreational and therefore therapeutic. They themselves continued to steer the treatment. Even now that dance-movement therapy is coming of age, the heads of many treatment teams ignore or fail to exploit the insights gathered by the adjunctive dance-movement therapist, simply because they are more comfortable with their own form of intervention. On the other side of the spectrum, many dance-movement therapists assume they are doing primary therapy because they are working individually. Misunderstandings permeate the professional milieu. Because of these misunderstandings, the clients frequently have to return to their primary therapist before they are ready to do so. Treatment is interrupted at an inorganic point when dance-movement therapist and client are still emotionally hooked into each other

Thus, the interpersonal and transferential aspects of the relationship can never be clarified and become integrated for either partner in the treatment dyad. Dance-movement therapists are also effectively prevented from evolving a consistent theory for interpretation. At this time, there is no theory or theoretical model, for interpretation within dance-movement therapy. Nevertheless, there appears to be agreement among those dance-movement therapists who work in an in-depth mode that such a model is a necessity (Dosamantes-Alperson, 1973-74, 1977, 1978; Whitehouse, 1977; Sandel, 1978, 1979, 1981; Bernstein, 1979, Espenak, 1981).

THERAPY IS A TWO-WAY STREET

The faculty of knowing one's life history emotionally and intellectually is the outcome of successful therapy. This applies to both partners in the treatment dyad, client and therapist. Where the client's cognitive activity stops, the therapist's interpretive activity first clarifies and then helps resolve the block toward further growth and evolution. This, too, is a two-way street. With each empathetically offered verbal or nonverbal interpretation, the therapist expands his or her own boundaries of knowing and feeling (Kris, 1956). The emphasis here, as in all effective treatment situations, is on empathy that has reached the level of full awareness so that it can be verbalized.

There are ex-clients of dance-movement therapists who claim that the good they derived from their interaction with their therapist resided in the therapist's "not getting into their heads" or "leaving their minds alone" (Greenberg, 1973, p. 227). Within the frame of reference presented here, these statements can be seen as manifestations of a resistance against recognizing how very important the interaction with the dance-movement therapist had become. Without the clarifying aspect of the interpretive action by the therapist, the strong feelings behind such statements were left to profilerate, to destroy the treatment situation.

One needs to have one's therapist in one's head if one wishes to identify with him or her. Leaving the therapist outside one's head means one hasn't internalized sufficiently, or dreads that the internalization will lead to self and other destruction.

It was Chace (1968) who used the phrase "Basic Dance" to describe the form of nonverbal communication acutely mentally ill people frequently employ. She saw this Basic Dance as the "externalization of inner feelings which cannot be expressed in rational speech but can only be shared in rhythmic, symbolic action" (p. 203). Because this is often the only form of communication left to such very ill people, Chace advocated Basic Dance as an Adjunctive Therapy. For many in the field, their responsibilities have taken them far beyond these initial phases as adjunct therapists despite the incompleteness of the Chace approach.

The spectacular early successes of dance therapy as adjunctive therapy seem indeed to have rested on Chace's discovery that deeply regressed or undeveloped individuals are at a level at which their bodies speak for them. The case of Carlos corroborates her findings. He was a handsome youngster who received schooling and treatment in a day treatment facility. Carlos was a teenager who spent much of his time whirling in circles that were executed faster and became smaller in direct proportion to his inner agitation. Sometimes his teacher managed to stop him by stern commands. At other times, medication slowed him into lethargic concentricity. On occasion, he would hold his head in his hands and sigh deeply. When he felt somewhat more in touch with reality he revealed himself as an intelligent young man whose dark good looks fascinated some of his female classmates. It was difficult to determine whether he had received medication on any given day or not. His mother often "forgot" whether she had given him his daily dose and therefore administered either double the amount prescribed or nothing at all. The single social worker responsible for all the families whose children attended the institution was hard-pressed to find a solution for this unhappy state of affairs. In the meantime Carlos whirled, sometimes quickly, sometimes slowly, and warded off all attempts at contact.

When he was assigned to dance-movement therapy, this phenomenon was difficult to understand as Basic Dance, because its expressive component was not immediately apparent. There aren't many people who can pirouette with as much finesse as Carlos. But the famous Whirling Dervishes were said to reach states of ecstasy in their whirling. In pushing past the nausea and disorientation of constant spinning one can reach a point of stillness and calm that is utterly removed from others. Could it be, then, that Carlos not only was releasing tension by whirling, but was performing a Basic Dance meant to avoid contact with the world? When he was mirrored, Carlos didn't even notice his therapist was there, spinning with him. Therefore she edged closer to him and grabbed for his hands. With a start, he stopped, gave the all-important eye-contact and said curtly: "Cut that out."

Had his world been entered too quickly? Not so, said his teacher. After all, his comment had been appropriate, and had apparently been the first direct and meaningful words he had spoken for a long time. On the next meeting, the therapist said to Carlos; "I would like to spin with you." "Okay," he said, to everyone's suprise. Eventually Carlos the Whirling Dervish waited around for his therapist's appearance so he'd have a companion in his "dance." Later, when mutual trust had been established, a fast waltz was substituted. This step-by-step progress opened the way for Carlos' further learning. Instead of being a schizophrenic person who whirled about, he was now a schizophrenic person who didn't whirl. A symptom had been conquered, no more. Carlos' interpersonal relationships and much of his behavior remained deeply disturbed despite classic dance-therapy intervention.

Some of the younger children in the same institution could not bend their knees. They hardly ever ran in the playground and had difficulty negotiating stairs, although nothing was wrong organically. Not one of them could even crawl correctly. Some just lay down on their stomachs when they were asked to imitate crawling. Therefore a series of basic movements, as opposed to Basic Dance, were instituted. They were asked to roll from side to side, or to stretch out on their tummies, and lift up their heads again and again in time to very slow classic music.

These sessions had more the flavor of a pre-gymnastic group. The question arose: Wasn't so much structure an imposition on these young clients, wasn't their creativity being stifled? The answer is obvious: it is hardly possible to be creative when one doesn't have the bodily tools for the expression of creativity.

***

Primary Means In-Depth

In facing the unconscious, primary dance-movement therapy as an in-depth approach is no different from other therapies. It merely employs a different human property, motility, as the means for reaching its goal.

That dance-movement therapy is becoming an in-depth therapy is attested to not only by the fact that more individuals present themselves for such intervention either through referral or on their own account, but also by the fact that in this writer's private practive, for instance, there has been a shift away from the deeply disturbed individual who was sent by another therapist for tension release, toward people who wish for the total form of intervention that integration of the body and mind can be. As many dance-movement therapists abandon the merely aesthetic and come to grips with what is useful and growth-producing (Schoop, 1971; Espenak, 1973; Schmais, 1974; Kalish, 1974; Bernstein, 1979) predictability has entered the field. It has been recognized that human motility undergoes change as the individual grows and matures (Mittelman, 1955, 1957; Kestenberg, 1967; Gesell, 1973; Siegel, 1973). If one links the observable movement patterns of an individual to developmental levels, an accurate statement can be made as to the fixation point when growth was first inhibited under the impact of trauma.

For example, if a grown man habitually employs the body stance of a toddler, with abdomen thrust forward and inability to rotate his pelvis, one may look for further evidence of trouble in the anal phase of psychosexual development, in the absence of freely given verbal associations and in the withholding of emotion.

The Aesthetic Mode In Dance-Movement Therapy

Given the origins in the aesthetics of dance there is often a temptation to overemphasize this aspect in treatment. Working only in the aesthetic mode can also establish harmony at least temporarily without theoretical structure. This type of intervention certainly does provide a coming-together of felt experiences, imagining and acting, but these integrations do not necessarily fortify the client through the next stressful life situation.

THE CASE OF BERNARD

A young man of high school age, Bernard, was assigned to dance-movement therapy because his teacher observed that he had an unusual facility for picking up rhythms heard on the radio or even in the speech of others. His diagnosis of ''elective mutism'' decribed a symptom but did not encompass developmental facets of his pathology. Bernard was known to be the son of a schizophrenic mother. After her death he was placed in the custody of a foster mother who later became alcoholic. When this second mother began to deteriorate, Bernard's despair knew no bounds. He began to curse and swear, to beat the woman and to comport himself in every way as potential murderer. The foster mother had to be hospitalized, and since there was no one to care for him, so was Bernard. When he and his foster mother were able to rejoin each other, Bernard had become a mute. No amount of cajoling, or behavior modification, or chemotherapy, had induced him to speak.

He was a dance therapist's dream come true, one might have thought. He could dance any situation, symbolize in movement any emotion at will. Unfortunately, there was always a contrived, stagey quality to his productions, so that one knew he was either teasing or just acting on what he thought was wanted of him. His feelings had not engaged his action. It was as though he were always watching himself and others from a distance. His own favorites were calypso rhythms and reggae.

He was seen twice a week. No other therapist worked with him at the time. Bernard immediately proceeded to make his therapist, this writer, uncomfortable, and himself comfortable, by choosing a rock record to dance to. He chose an Elton John selection, *Crocodile Rock*. All attempts to contact him or to join his dance, were either warded off or ignored. As time went on, he stopped turning away from me and danced with me or, rather, he allowed me to dance with him. Whenever a comment was made like ''I think you are comfortable being silent,'' or ''Perhaps you prefer being silent,'' he would smirk.

In the third month of dancing to *Crocodile Rock* twice a week, he began to nod ''Hello'' when I said ''Hello.'' He managed to produce countertransferential agony that attacked my image of myself as a competent dance-movement therapist. Pressure was mounting from the treatment team to accomplish something. Everybody knew that Bernard could move like an angel. What therefore, was he doing in dance-movement therapy? Movement was *not* one of his deficit areas. I tried to keep my agitation out of my movements as we went about out ritualistic *Crocodile Rock*. Every once in a while, and usually just when I was ready to scream, Bernard would either wink at me or give me a brilliant smile. I began to feel as though I were a fish being played on a hook. I managed to keep calm, however, and, along with meek efforts at verbalizations, mirrored Bernard's sleek movements. They had the easy, somewhat sardonic quality of a junior hustler, and brought the city ghettos into the treatment room. Eventually I even began to enjoy the proceedings. I noticed that my own movements took on some of the same sleekness when dancing with Bernard. Week after week, he dutifully did his warm-ups, improvised on themes set by me, and regularly turned to his *Crocodile Rock*. Eventually, dancing to this was the only activity we indulged in together.

Some six months later came the beginning of a breakthrough. Bernard was expansive in that he acknowledged his therapist's presence with a smile. Very deliberately, he swaggered over to the record player and selected *Honky Cat*, also by Elton John. We danced vigorously once more and again I tried my interpretive arts. I knew that the selection of new music signified something of a turning point. But how could I acknowledge that I understood and approved, besides accepting his dance? At the end, Bernard took over. He reached out his hand in the ''give me five'' gestural jargon of his environment. I speedily gave the expected handclasp and was rewarded by the first mumbled words: ''Funky Honky Siegel.'' Frantically trying to cope with tears that invaded my eyes, I searched for an answer that would acknowledge the transferential aspect of our budding relationship within a context that Bernard could accept. If I were funky and honky, what was he? Was he saying: Don't come so close, lady, you might swallow me? Or was the message simply, ''I can talk to you now because you accepted, and joined my silence.'' Quickly, I decided that it was most important to reaffirm Bernard's selfhood. ''Cool Cat Bernard?'' I offered.

He was delighted. This was the turning point, indeed. Bernard's dances now became stately minuets, enacted with a minimum of contact between us. We touched fingertips only and walked slowly together; or, facing each other, we would sway in a waltz while Bernard told me of the savagery that had destroyed his life. Eventually, he began to talk to teachers and others as well. Later, unfortunately, events in his life were too overpowering for him to handle. His guardians removed him from the setting in which he was beginning to blossom. He was hospitalized again, and when he reappeared, there were only vestiges of his exuberance and beauty of movement left.

I learned an important lesson from Bernard. Although many growth-producing sessions had occurred, and his body and mind were indeed able to express harmoniously, with fluency and most creatively, what it was he needed and wanted, the interaction had not been long enough, nor in-depth enough to provide him with a bulwark against the overwhelming brutality in his environment. Interestingly, incidentally, the loose-jointed beauty of his earlier dancing disappeared when he began to tell the tale of his life history. As some of his cognitive functions expanded, deep depression surfaced and engulfed the qualitative aspects of his movements. This is not suprising when on e examines the dyamics of depression. Bernard had experienced so many losses and so many disappointments that part of his selfhood had been lost. He could no longer mourn but had to punish himself cruelly with self-reproaches and maniacal punishment fantasies (Freud, 1917). The aesthetics of the interaction had allowed Bernard to make contact and to reach a level on which a permanent change could have effected if his environment had been supportive of his therapy, and if his therapist had known how to engage him in a productive way.

***

DANCE TRAINING
REMAINS IMPORTANT[1]

It can be seen how important the dance forms were in the early stages of many treatments. But among the different approaches to dance-movement therapy some seem to negate the need for thorough dance training. This is not so in the psychoanalytic frame of reference presented here. Dance training remains the important college through which one must pass in order to acquire the skills for graduate training. A psychoanalyst must personally have experienced the emergence of the self in his own analysis in order to be an informed and empathetic guide for the analysands' struggles in the labyrinth of the unconscious.

In just this manner, a dance-movement therapist must have explored the netherlands of her movement possibilities. This is not possible without thorough dance training. Thorough training means that one has mastered several techniques in an anatomically correct way and that these techniques have become a component of one's personal movement repertoire. This *has* to take place before one can respond immediately on both symbolic and conscious levels to the movement of another, such as a patient. Supervising interns for their practica in dance-movement therapy confirms this point of view. Those who do not think of themselves as dancers are many times bright, intuitive, and resourceful, but they are psychotherapists who also use movement, rather than dance-movement therapists. Therefore, they do not know how to complete a movement phrase or how to connect a Basic Dance to a dance form. It seems ironic that these bright, young, intuitive persons who say of themselves that they are "organic movers," can identify psychologic structures but cannot identify a pavane or dance a minuet. But it is these dance forms and styles which provide the bridge between unconscious movement emanations and the conscious aesthetic experience.

---

[1]The American Dance Therapy Association published requirements for registry in 1972.

TOWARD A THEORY OF PSYCHOANALYTIC
DANCE-MOVEMENT THERAPY

The intellectualization of dance-movement therapy began, not surprisingly, when attempts at conceptualizations were made. It was postulated that movement per se reflects personality, that interpersonal relationships established through movement with the client support and produce changes in functioning, and that significant changes occur on the movement level that may affect the total personality. Psyche and soma are seen as continuously interactive (Schmais, 1974).

Trudie Schoop, a pioneer dance therapist, wrote in 1971: ". . .where psycho-analysis brings about change in the mental attitude, there should be a corresponding change in physical behavior. When a dance therapist brings about a change in body behavior, there should be a corresponding change in the mind. Both methods want to change the total being, body and mind"(p. 5.).

This holistic approach to the human being is a major concern in all forms of dance movement therapy (Berstein, 1979). After all, we live in, with, and through our bodies, and contact all of life's tasks through bodily means.

Missing in these conceptualizations are consistent theoretical structures that deal with defense and transferences. This book attempts to address these problems.

The use of psychoananlytic language was spurred not only by the fact that many professionals knew it already, but also by this writer's additional training in psychoanalytic psychotherapy. I sought this additional training because there were so many questions unanswered in dance therapy, as is outlined above.

Along with others, I began to call myself a dance-movement therapist, because many of my early clients were not capable of Basic Dance. Their activities did not include the process of creating a dance with symbolic content. Rather, they had to learn some of the movement activities that are acquired as a matter of course and with ease by someone whose development and maturation is not impeded. The medium that made it possible for these clients to acquire these rudiments for living were the tenuous interpersonal relationships, known in psychoanalytic language as part object relationships, that they formed with their therapist. Because I usually employ recorded music or vocal sounds to help structure the sessions, the uninitiated might think that there is a dancelike quality to these beginning movement experiences, but emotion connected to movement does not come into play until higher developmental levels have been reached. To begin with, feelings, sensations, and movement are random, fragmented, and unstructured. So, including "movement" as a descriptive addition seemed appropriate.

MOTILITY AND THE EGO

Perhaps it would be good to define the word "ego" as it is used here first. When I speak of someone's ego, I do not mean that he is conceited nor do I subscribe to it as a theoretical construct only.

Freud himself never used the word *ego*. He always said and wrote *ich*, which literally translated means "I." Therefore, his concept *Körper-ich* (body ego) means the body-I, or I-the-body. This comes very close to the ideal envisioned for dance-movement therapy. If one substitutes the word "I" for "ego" in all of Freud's translated writings, an immediacy of perception results for the reader which negates the popular misconception of Freudian thought as removed and cold.

In 1923 Freud moved away from the use of the *ich* as connoting the entire mental self, to his structural theory. He divided the mental self into the well-known major components, id, ego, and superego. The most important task of the ego in this construct is its job of mediating between inner strivings and outer demands. Freud saw the ego evolving out of the undifferentiated potentialities given at birth through the medium of the object relations.

The "I" arises out of the matrix of nondifferentiation, out of understanding neither "I" nor Non-I, inner or outer. But this "I" in dance-movement therapy is always, and foremost, the bodily "I" with which we touch, see, feel, hear, smell, and construct our reality. There is no activity that is alive which is not of the body. Thus, the construct Ego which mediates between inner and outer strivings, and reaches its antennae into both the unconscious and the conscious, is also the entire self in this form of therapy.

OBJECT RELATIONSHIPS

The word *object* in this context means "an emotionally significant person." The choice of terminology is somewhat unfortunate because many people think of an "object" as a concrete, usually inanimate thing. Nevertheless, object relations and object-relations theory in psychoanalytic language mean one's relationships with emotionally important people who had, or have, influence on one's life. This object relationship, as all other human functions and attributes, is seen to undergo wide-ranging changes in the evolutionary process from birth to death. Some of these changes are known to be predictable occurrences in the lives of all humans (Mittelman, 1955, 1957; Spitz, 1965; Mahler, 1968; Gesell, 1972; and Siegel, 1973). Age-specific maturational and developmental phases which overlap, take place. Most commonly, these are designated to be the oral, anal, and genital phases, each with its specific hallmarks. We carry with us the resolutions and conclusions we have come to in each phase into the next one, so that vestiges of all of our life's experiences are always with us, whether we consciously acknowledge them or not.

The transitional stages between phases are seen as particularly vulnerable to trauma because old ways of adaptation are felt to be no longer adequate, while new ones are not yet firmly in place (Hartmann, 1937, Kris, 1952, Spitz, 1965). For example, a toddler may have learned from experience that mother will reappear in time to provide food, and thus be free from anxiety about her absence until mealtime. If something delays her, nothing in life has prepared the young child for the thought-processes available to an adult, i.e., the toddler cannot yet rationalize that she may have been delayed for reasons not of her choosing. If mother often does not reappear on time, and does not reassure her child after her return, the toddler may decide that she had deserted him or her and give himself over to depression and feelings of abandonment (Spitz 1965). Should such an untoward chain of events be repeated too often, fear of abandonment and an inability to trust loved persons may be carried into adult life.

This is an oversimplification, of course, but it does point toward the kind of thinking most Developmentalists, such as this writer, prefer. Further, Spitz and others have shown that if any one human agency is prevented from maturing in an age-adequate way by either psychologic or organic factors, deviant adaptations to life will result. This "deviance" may be a relatively minor obstacle to full freedom of locomotion, as in not being a good social dancer, or may be an important inability to move about in a consciously directed way at all.

When one acquaints oneself with the specific human agencies that can be expected to come to light in any given developmental phase, one can look at an individual and literally see in what phase he or she may have gotten stuck, or where a person's fixation point may be. The higher up the developmental ladder an individual has climbed, the more complex this becomes. "Seeing" or diagnosing many factors in both the person and the environment is necessary (A. Freud, 1965). Nevertheless, the fixation point, the place where trauma overtook development and partially halted it, can most often be ascertained. The claim of dance-movement therapy is that it can also be ascertained in motility. This volume is written from that point of view.

A word of explanation is in order once again. By higher or lower developmental levels, no value-judgment of any kind is implied. My clients have taught me to respect the strength it has taken most of them to exist at all. The most deeply impaired among them are frequently those who have fought most valiantly just to stay alive. Therefore, I try not to view human behavior as good or bad, but as merely existing. The labeling that is an inevitable concomitant of ordering phenomena is not intended to carry with it pejorative connotations; it is intended to produce clarity among a wealth of materials.

The section on *Transference and Countertransference* addresses itself to the idea that these feeling-states take on a somewhat different meaning in this form of intervention, although they deal with the same phenomena as are experienced in other therapies. Because the entire body, not only part of it, is the medium for therapy, dance-movement therapists experience more direct echoes of a client's feeling state in their own physical and total self. Analysts speak of "resonating with the client" (Greenson, 1967) but, by and large, their bodily sensations as a countertransferential component are not included in their conscious use of these feelings. Notable exceptions are Reich (1933), Schafer (1953) and Jacobs (1973). Those courageous souls, who acknowledge and use their counter-transference as a treatment tool, nevertheless rarely get around to stating clearly what parts of their bodies heralded the emergence of what feeling state. (Searles, 1965; LeBoit and Capponi, 1979). For the dance-movement therapist, depending on the depth of insight attained, repeated physical symptoms signal countertransferential phenomena. Interns always seem to have headaches, an understandable reaction to the overwhelming stimulus of being with a client or clients for the first time. Body sensations become more identifiable with experience, and experienced dance-movement therapists learn how to accept and integrate them.

CATHEXIS

Translators have had difficulties with transmitting all of Freud's thoughts accurately from one language to the other. Sometimes, personal biases were involved, at other times there simply wasn't an adequate English word around. Therefore, Brill (1944) coined the word *cathexis* when he translated Freud's works. It means "emotional charge" of a body part or a mental process so that it is especially prominent in awareness. In dance-movement therapy, we are always dealing with body tensions and body parts, especially cathected movement patterns or decathected parts of the body. For instance, in certain atypical children and adults, the skin surface may be so decathected that they must injure themselves in order to feel at all. Others cathect their pelvis, or their breathing apparatus to such an extent that hips and pelvic region or the lungs become the major focus of their emotional lives. The hope is that these statements will provide a guide for what is to follow. It would be gratifying to have more answers. Until more are found, here are hypotheses that emerged during nearly 20 years of using dance-movement therapy as an in-depth, primary tool.

Chapter 1

THE UNITY OF
BODY AND MIND

There are many parallels to ego-psychoanalytic thinking in the sort of dance-movement therapy described here. Schilder (1950) believed that our body images are "the crystalization of our lives' experiences." Dance-movement therapists operate under the assumption that movement reflects personality (Schmais, 1974). These formulations from different disciplines state that our modes of locomoting and carrying our bodies have specific meaning and are formed by acceptance or rejection of both inner and outer stimuli as well as by conscious and unconscious perceptions.

Particularly striking is the emphasis of some psychoanalysts on the unity or continuum between body and mind. For Freud (1933) the body held all sources of consciousness. Hoffer (1949) described the earliest formation of a rudimentary body ego. Fenichel (1945) speaks of "disturbances of inner sensitivity and body feelings" (p. 248). Schilder maintains that "there is a close interrelation between muscular sequences and inner attitude so that not only does the inner attitude connect up with muscular states, but also every sequence

17

of tensions and relaxations provokes a specific attitude. When there is a specific motor sequence it changes the inner situation and even provokes a different muscular sequence''(p. 208).

Thinking from this point of view allows one to speak about essentially nonverbal intersubjective communications between clients and therapist in a more objective way. The psychoanalytic theoreticians cited present a framework of thought in which the interactivity between body and mind was self-evident. Following them, the ubiquitous split between psyche and soma can be seen as culturally induced and often traumatically underscored even in relatively unimpaired people. In working with bodily manifestations, a distinction must be made between catharsis and abreaction. In a true catharsis people no longer know how or why they are functioning. They are consumed by the released discharge of pent-up emotions from the past. They rarely have a recollection of what it is they did while catharting. Abreaction, on the other hand, does not go this far. Clients have to be encouraged ''to feel their feelings'' and to observe themselves while doing so. The client will still cry, or scream, or withdraw, but be aware of doing so, of being the one who is experiencing. Thus, the uncontrolled aspects of catharsis becomes harnessed to the ego.

The physical sense of well-being that follows when an inappropriate movement pattern is abandoned keeps the client slugging toward the goal and often helps overcome resistances when verbalization and interpretation fail.

In other words: intellectualization as a defensive function, and splitting not only of the ego but of the inner and outer person, and warding off of affect are as clearly visible on a muscularly expressed basis as in their psychic counterpart.

Dancing as communal ritual and approved channel for abreaction has long been with us. War dances to build the individual's rage to a fever pitch and to reinforce it by fusion with his like-minded brethren, religious ecstasy to the point of self-hypnosis by the Dervishes and the Isawa of North Africa, the Rock and Roll of our own culture with its displayed but futile sexuality (Wow—look at me trip, but don't touch. I'll do that by myself), all point to the human need to experience oneself somatically.

In psychoanalytically oriented dance-movement therapy, it is possible to re-establish through dancelike movements the harmony that existed prior to splitting and repression and to satisfy the need for somatic experience.

BEGINNING CONCEPTUALIZATIONS

Six basic working hypotheses emerged out of doing dance-movement therapy within a psychoanalytic framework. Their consistent application produced predictability and demonstrated that dance-movement therapy could be used as a primary, in-depth tool. They are:

1. Concern for recreating the harmonious whole of psyche and soma by extending help toward more adequate physical functioning and through building a better body image;
2. Acceptance of catharsis as part of the process of regression toward the fixation point;
3. Insights gained by observation are employed in the working-through process;
4. Preferred patterns of movement are integrated into the sessions as a starting point for specifically choreographed dances and individually designed exercises;
5. Improvisations are welcomed as steppingstones towards autonomous functioning;
6. Skeletomuscular inhibitions are seen as an attempt to express and control aggressive impulses.

These points parallel the classic psychoanalytic concept of symptom-formation as a compromise between defensive function and the need to express the repressed.

In applying these concepts other psychoanalytic parallels

and concerns came into focus as well. A major one in this body-oriented work was

DESOMATIZATION

A besetting worry of psychoanalytically oriented teachers and psychologists is their assumption that by dealing so directly with the body, dance-movement therapy might encourage rather than discourage primary process thinking and acting out. Why would a person whose thoughts are dominated by irrational, primitive wishes that lead into stormy and erratic behavior become calmer and more self-contained after a movement session, they ask. Wouldn't it be too stimulating, not to say sexual, to dance with a person the client likes?

The answer could be a simple one. When a client who is stuck in early developmental phases, or has regressed to them, is given an opportunity to release tension in movement, this person can begin to form clearer perceptions of the world. When symbolic condensations and displacement find their movement resolution, it is safe to give them up, and to let reality in. Schilder states that each sensation holds its own motor answer. Therefore, if a schizophrenic feels an alien sensation in the hand as though it were floating overhead in space, she or he may deny possessing a hand and refuse to touch anything; or may merrily chase after this hand-shaped thing as though it were a butterfly. In dance-movement therapy sessions it is easy to demonstrate that hands are attached to arms by stroking them and then swinging them. Following this stroking the client may then wish to investigate if the therapist too has hands and arms that are similarly connected. Sometimes this is followed by a joyous period of playing with arms and hands, like small children who are discovering their body parts. The need to chase a body part fantasied lost diminishes in direct proportion to the growing knowledge: this is my arm and this is my hand. But before such direct body-image building can take place, it is often necessary to dance vigorously without any other purpose than to draw off tension.

About clients who function on a more evolved plane, other questions arise.

How does dancing, for instance, help an inhibited person to reach her or his potential and what do breathing exercises and individual improvisation and relaxation techniques have to do with an individual's psychic development?

Schur (1955) in his *Comments on the Metapsychology of Somatization* informs us that:

> From (this) undifferentiated state maturation proceeds in several directions. One, for example, is the development of coordinated muscle function. Another is the maturation of the mental apparatus. There is a parallel of development, and mutual interdependence, between the maturation of the central nervous system and the motor apparatus, the stabilization of homeostatic processes . . . as an essential part of ego-formation. All this results in an increasing desomatization to reactions to certain excitations. The development tends toward . . . replacement of action by thought and reduction of vegetative discharge phenomena (p. 122-123).

Schur's *Comments* are quite simply the statement that maturation brings desomatization with it. Instead of acting on each sensation, perception or thought-dictates of inner and outer needs are selectively followed. When this process fails, *re*somatization, or a physiologic regression occurs. Schur maintains that a physiologic regression is a preverbal, pre-ego state which is said to play a major role in psychosomatic disorders such as ulcerative colitis, asthma, some forms of hypertension and so on. These disorders have also been called "anxiety equivalents" (Fenichel). Or, to phrase it differently, even when there is no awareness of anxiety, somatization takes place but energy is discharged inwardly, similarly to the way a neonate discharges energies silently inward until that point in development when skin surfaces become known entities through the ministrations of the mother (Jacobson, 1964).

Somatization takes place throughout the entire range of the nosologic categories. It is in this area of somatization that the movement and dance therapist can be of help.

Where Schur says that there is a parallel development and mutual interdependence between psychological and biological processes, the movement and dance therapist points out that psyche and soma are essentially one, we live within and through our bodies. Nevertheless, speech as expression and as communication has to be included in order to round out and complete the picture. The result of working within a theoretical framework was a dissolution of the preoccupation with the dance product of clients, and created the leisure of stillness as clients began to talk about their life histories and daily occurrences. But speech is also a tension release.

Speech Is Tension Release

Listening to clients' needs includes looking at posture and gesture, breathing patterns and tone of voice, rhythms and tensions that are alway present when a client either reveals something or hides in speech and in movement. Talking as a tension release makes catharsis less necessary. While moving or creating dance, it was no longer hard to find a theme. The clients' lives provided the theme.

An asthmatic woman had been taught to breathe deeply in many therapeutic sessions but was still plagued by her illness. We had to talk to each other for a long time before she was willing to give up the idea that her illness was "merely" physiologic. Breathing exercises culled from both Yoga and another dance-movement therapist's intervention brought her relief. But the chronic tensions and cramping in her chest did not leave her until she had allowed herself to trust me enough to scream in my presence and to tell sobbingly that her mother had never come to comfort her when she was frightened as a child at night. Her improvisations were not meaningful to her and did not connect with her feelings until she could see her present therapist as someone who could be called at night when the distress was acute. This does not mean that all clients are invited to call any time they are uncomfortable. This sort of leaning against the therapist is accepted only when the developmental level of the client demands the presence of a nurturing person.

FOSTERING AUTONOMY

Such episodes raised key theoretical questions. Wasn't there the possibility that so much nurturance also curtailed the client's independent functioning? This is a point upon which psychoanalysts have argued since their discipline's inception. Freud (1914) warned against overgratifying clients. When a need is fulfilled, it disappears from consciousness and can no longer be explored. Therefore it is important to find just the right balance in bringing clients' hidden wishes and conflicts to the surface and then examining them while they are available.

Hunger disppears when one eats. This is true of emotional hunger also. If one has always yearned for a loving friend why find one in reality if the therapist fills that role? In my early days as a therapist I found it difficult to refuse an invitation to a birthday party which I had heard so much about from my client; and I would really have liked to have been present when another one married. But I could not be the fairy godmother the birthday child longed for. My presence would simply have reinforced her idea that if she pleaded long enough and hard enough she could manipulate anyone into doing anything, as she did her family, and in school. The bride needed a stand-in mother, one that was more attractive and giving than her own. Her therapist's appearance at that wedding would have contributed to the vengeful feelings of a young woman who despised her own mother.

Clients have to find their solutions themselves while being securely cradled by the therapist's certainty that their distress can be worked through. Their therapist's presence at their festive gatherings would have made them feel good, so good, in fact, that further work on their conflicts would have been more difficult.

Freud and his followers have evoked storms of protest from needy patients who have felt pushed aside, and from indignant humanitarians who thought sufferers were further tortured on the couch by the supposed emotional unavailability of the analyst. In actuality the dilemma lies in finding the right balance between being merely a mirror for the client, and providing the certainty of the therapist's availability at the same time. The emotional position vis-a-vis clients has to be both distant and close, i.e., *understanding* is always shared, rarely emotions. This does not mean that I feel nothing. Rather, experience has taught me that Freud was right. Clients do not need the extra burden of their therapist's feelings. They need a guide to untangle their own difficulties and the freedom to experience their therapist in whatever form they wish. At the same time, feelings about a client inform the interpretive actions chosen. These interpretive actions may relate to the present or the past.

FREE ASSOCIATION AND IMPROVISATION

Eruptions from the past can be seen with particular clarity in movement. Psychotic clients, for instance, are hardly ever able to improvise at length in synchronicity with their therapist. Improvising is closely related to free association in psychoanalysis. Both techniques are designed to tap the unconscious. While improvising in a safe situation, neurotics may reveal an important fact or fantasy about past relationships in the way they either try to draw the therapist into their productions, or ignore, insult, provoke, or implore the therapist by their conscious expressive gestures. Example after example of the transference relationships expressed in movement come to mind.

A woman always danced with her back to the therapist and became acutely uncomfortable the moment she faced her. After a while she discovered that the therapist reminded her of her mother who preferred boys and thought vaginas were shameful. Another woman regularly placed herself as far away from the therapist as possible, looked down, and confined all her activities to the smallest amount of space which still permitted her to move. With some amazement, the therapist found herself perceived as a teaching nun in this client's transferential constellation. It seemed that in her particular religious school, small, ladylike gestures and downcast eyes won approval from the nuns who instructed the little girls. Men often need to show that they are much stronger than their therapist because they do not ever want to become dependent as they were once dependent on their mothers.

With psychotic clients the situation becomes even more directly expressive of their needs and their developmental level. One needs to be careful about when and how to allow improvisations. Because improvisation taps the unconscious, psychotic people may easily become lost in the labyrinth of their own imagining and frighten themselves with the feelings that come up when they act as though they were their own hallucinations. The "as-if" quality that underlies even the strongest emotional expression from a neurotic can turn into a frightening encounter with imagined demons in someone who can no longer distinguish reality from fantasy. The imagistic experience can be so overpowering for schizophrenic people that they cannot find their way back into reality.

This was brought home in particular when working with an adolescent, Maida, whose diagnosis was said to include some paranoid features. She seemed to be a good candidate for dance-movement therapy. Her ability to express in movement what she felt had the immediacy as well as the clearly defined distance of a fine theatrical performance. She also relished the good feelings that she derived from her own grandiose gestures and high leaps. Breathing exercises always brought her down from any excitation she might have experienced during the session.

What the dance-movement techniques did not manage to accomplish was a reconnection with reality. She had learned only too well that being quiet was mistaken for acquienscence by her surroundings. So she would leave her sessions physically quiet but mentally engrossed in her hallucinations. Her illusory persecutors in the form of huge eyes that hung menacingly above her in a red sky never left her. What she shared with her therapist was merely an attempt to catch and destroy these menaces, along with some talk about eyes. She expressed this by jumping and leaping like a ballet dancer in *grands jetés* and using her arms like a hunter who wishes to catch birds in a large net. Her movements were always fully connected and fluid and never showed the jerkiness other psychotic people exhibit. She told differing stories in conjunction with similar improvisations so that her tension releases were also an enactment of her fantasy. The monotonous similarity of her dances aroused her therapist's doubts and led to further investigation. Maida was unable to take a step back into reality until more structured sessions were offered. Then she conquered her persecution fears under the guidance of a positive transference. This is only one of many examples which show that to assign meaning to any posture or gesture or dance is futile unless a great deal is known about the client involved.

THE NEED FOR CLARITY

In working with people like Maida, it is particularly important to achieve clarity. Of course, that's often a difficult feat.

Especially in groups, all sorts of uncalled-for happenings can take place when meanings of movements have not been clarified and grounded in reality. For instance, during a long and arduous period of treatment with some acting-out teenagers who had been in trouble with the police, this therapist was less careful than she should have been with potentially dangerous results. Although aware that all of these kids carried the word "schizophrenia" on their diagnostic charts, they performed in such a nearly normal and expressive way that the therapist temporarily lost her guard, and they their connection to reality, even though all were moving appropriately and fluidly.

The incident in question occurred during the second year of regular twice-weekly meetings. The group had advanced into a place where the issues of trust could be examined. Anger at probation officers, teachers, social wokers, and the therapist had been talked about, staged in mini-psychodramas, and even in a specifically choreographed dance.

The movement interaction now included an old "trust game." The group stood in a circle, shoulder to shoulder, while one person would stand stiffly in the middle and let him or herself fall against the nearest body in the circle who would then hand him or her on to the next. Generally it makes good sense for the therapist *not* to join in because leader participation can contaminate the emerging group dynamics in such activity, but because this group seemed to have such a need to see their therapist as one of their own, she complied. For them, this wish was developmentally sound. It worked fine. Participants were full of wonder that their "old lady" was not afraid and was "cool" like themselves. Somebody even managed to point out that "old lady" could mean a person's "girlfriend" and everyone nearly choked with laughter that their therapist could possibly be anyone's girlfriend.

From there the group progressed to lifting each other. One person would lie down stiffly on the floor while everone else would gently lift and then rock him or her. All looked forward to this exercise because it allowed expressions of tender feelings for each other. The lifted person could request being rocked, or being sung to without fear that he was seen as "mushy" by the group. The lifted person was always placed straight upright upon descent in order to facilitate clear connections with the floor and reality.

One day the group decided that they would like to give their therapist something good after all had agreed that being lifted was like flying. She was duly lifted and gently cradled, but had enough sense to look at the direction in which the bearers were carrying her. Panic hit when I realized that the intent was to truly make me fly—out the window! Struggles and screams brought teachers and aides running to block the group's intent. However, the boys were absolutely furious that I had not trusted them enough to give me this good experience. They simply would not believe that I would have been badly hurt had they made me fly out the window. "But you are our old lady " they said, "we wouldn't hurt you." The next two months were spent with filling balloons with water and air and dropping them out of the window in order to demonstrate that soft things full of fluid, like bodies, splash and split when thrown out of the window.

This incident illustrates that deeply regressed clients may first have to have reality testing reinforced by activities such as tracing the outline of their own body while listening to soothing music, or to discover that the room is safe. They need another chance to live through the body-image building stages of the earliest mother-child dyad. The therapist has to offer herself as a "second-chance" mother to someone who is on that developmental level. Moving and dancing and talking together build external and internal structure until the grown-up baby-client can give up dependency and can go on to the individuation-separation phase.

NEUTRALITY AS A THERAPEUTIC TOOL

Neurotic clients are encouraged to move by themselves once they have acquired a movement repertoire of their own. If they wish to include the therapist in their dances, they do so by dancing around her, touching the wall and floor in back and under her or by insisting that they need company in their dances. It would be a fatal error to superimpose the therapist's movement repertoire on a client who no longer needs a model.

In this way, the neutrality that psychoanalysts speak of is also established. Of necessity the neutrality a dance-movement therapist maintains has a different quality than that of a therapist who is not visible to the client, as the psychoanalyst is not visible to the analysand on the couch. The closest parallel would be to the child analyst who watches the child-client play. Some of the more sophisticated clients have teasingly likened this mode of being with them as "play therapy for adults."

They might be right. There is a lot of laughter in the later stages of the therapeutic discoveries together after defenses have been loosened.

DEFENSES

Defenses and their function are another concept familiar to both psychoanalysts and dance-movement therapists. Once clients drop their particular pattern of defending themselves, recovery of memory, more correct physical placement and alleviation of symptoms follow both in psychoanalysis and in dance-movement therapy, if the therapist of either persuasion has recognized anxiety as defensive and has lent his or her ego to that of the patient.

The struggle to bring the defenses out into the open can precipitate a strong resistance in the client. It is essential to recognize that defenses also serve an adaptive function (Hartmann, 1958). Clients breath in a shallow fashion or hold their backs rigidly because this once helped them through a traumatic situation which they had been unable to resolve. To meet strong defenses head-on produces anxiety and may even propel a client right out of therapy for good. In fact, quite a few clients show up for dance-movement therapy because they hope to avoid confrontation with the unconscious. They refuse to ac-cept that their behavior might be in part controlled by something that can be neither measured, weighed, nor seen. To point out to such a person that this very statement might indicate fear would be fatal to the therapy.

A dancer comes to mind who presented herself with one single large complaint which she felt was ruining her career. She had strangely shaped legs which looked knock-kneed. When she did her stretches on the floor, however, her legs looked straight and perfect. The minute she added the weight of her body in standing, the curious turning in took place without her volition. She had changed careers from ballet to modern dance and had even found a teacher who thought of classic turn-out in dancing as obscene. Nevertheless, Cerise could not control her legs enough to be performance-ready in the opinion of her teachers. Sometimes she managed to get parts in which she could hide under long skirts. Then, her perfomance quality was usually praised but her career never went further than dancing with small companies who were in need of fill-ins.

Cerise had undertaken a number of body-therapies and retraining courses all of which she reported to have temporarily given her control over those turned-in legs and knees. As soon as she had to perform, back she went to her old mode. There wasn't much one could give her in the way of movement that she didn't already know. But it was possible to work toward an awareness of the "inner woman." When Cerise achieved the ability to improvise without falling back on her extensive training, when she allowed an emotion to carry her through movement, she was asked how and why she had rocked and fallen to the floor like a child in a tantrum. In amazement she acknowledged that "something inside of me made me do it." The *woman* Cerise made her appearance inside of the *dancing-machine* Cerise only after a prolonged period of time, after many sessions in which her improvisations were marvelously acrobatic but without content. When she acknowledged the "something inside of her" Cerise's thighs and knees gave up their stranglehold on each other. She became able to turn them out from the hip socket. She observed this herself without interpretation or clarification from the therapist.

The defense which Cerise used most frequently was denial. She claimed to have no unconscious. Along with this went a disavowal of body feelings and the assumption that she could control her legs out of their peculiar position without acknowledging the expressive components of this position.

Defenses, and other psychoanalytic concepts, most often are developmentally organized.

DEVELOPMENTAL THEORY

Psychoanalysis as a developmental psychology offers an unprecedented diagnostic tool in its theory of maturational evolution which includes psychosexual phases, the various steps in object relationship, and physical maturation.

Each of the various developmental and maturational phases carries with it a general set of movement and muscular patterns, indicating levels of object relationships which, in turn, can alert the therapist of either persuasion toward what to expect in the ongoing treatment situation. This concept is elucidated in the table at the end of this chapter.

How does this look in the dance-movement therapy studio?

A client whose turn-out would be the envy of a classical dancer but who unfortunately locks the knees so tightly as to have to walk like a robot, or someone who cannot separate hip, torso, and head, but uses all three body parts as one unit, obviously is not very well acquainted with his or her body, possibly no more so than a toddler.

Toddlers are just learning that they can leave and then return to mother, that she will reappear after a lengthy shopping trip. In short, they are learning both about their body and about their love object, mother, and how far she can be trusted through the physical acitivity of coming and going. This is the "separation individuation" phase of development.

Once the therapist recognizes the "oral" level of the type of client described above, she must prepare herself to accept the clinging anxious behavior of such individuals and become the strong mother who literally teaches the toddler-patient, possibly of mature years, to locomote with less effort and to use the body in a fashion more appropriate to adult behavior. Such a client would most likely be psychotic and need a "real object," as opposed to the neurotic who is expected to use the therapist as a transference object only.

In analytic language, when doing dance-movement therapy, the ego of the psychotic client is strengthened by building the important ego function of walking which at the same time helps the client to perceive a small wedge of reality in the form of more organically placed walking. This in turn allows for renewed attempts by the psychotic to relate to another person without distortion. Object-related motor activity stimulates renewed attempts at body-image building and internalization of object representations.

Or, quite simply, by allowing the dance-movement therapist to help him or her walk more correctly, the psychotic is also saying "Yes, there is a possibility of loving and being loved since the person here really does not want to destroy me but is giving me something good."

Interpretation

Dance-movement therapists interpret nonverbally by mirroring, completing a movement phrase, or offering a second chance around. But unless the client is quite astonishingly intact, and can function like a choreographer of personal life history, verbal interpretation is also necessary, as has been mentioned. Permanent changes rarely happen without such talking. Examples and instances were cited in which clients made discoveries about themselves that led to insight and change. Sometimes the changes occur before the insight can be verbalized. For instance, Cerise began to be able to turn out from the hips before she understood that she had also been furious with her mother, and later her teachers, who wanted her to be modest. She eventually added childhood memories in which masturbation was forbidden. Her mother told her tales about children whose hands would rise up out of their graves if they "touched themselves there." Clearly, there was no way this level of understanding could have been reached if her behavior and verbalizations had not been interpreted. All clients, including the nonverbal ones, benefit from this mode.

In order to interpret, one needs to listen carefully to what a client says while looking carefully at what he or she does. After matching these data with what is already known about the client's history, one may come up with an interpretation. Optimally, a genetic proposition which is entirely based on the client's material can be included. Hartmann and Kris (1945) define genetic propositions as statements which "describe why, in a past situation of conflict a specific solution was adopted, why the one was retained, and the other dropped and what causal relations exist between these and later development"(p. 17). Quite simply, a genetic proposition is the result of a piece of detective work which explains infantile, or less mature behavior, in someone who has passed the age when the infantilism would have been appropriate. For instance, a toddler may have discovered that if she smiles prettily and gives a kiss to a new acquaintance, the adults around her will heartily applaud her. But if she goes about doing the same thing when she has become a young woman, people will call this same behavior impulsive, crazy, or inappropriate. The question of why she would want to conduct herself like this could be the focus of an interpretation. The aim is always to free the client for volitional action and to offer aid in casting off the shackles of the past.

In psychoanalytically oriented dance-movement therapy this aim is accomplished by paying equal attention to speech and motility. Not only emotional states and events but bodily behavior in relationship to these states are investigated. Thus, not only the inter- and intrasystemic workings of clients' psyches is interpreted but also as many aspects of their motility as they feel free to use.

Most members of the psychoanalytic community subscribe

to the idea that no true reshaping of the individual on any level can occur if the cognitive functions of the individual are not involved along with interpersonal happenings. However, psychoanalysts are opposed to interpretation as a tool among other therapeutic modalities. Some feel that by interpreting in the presence of "felt and concrete experience" in the treatment sessions through dance and movement, interpretation could concretize, rather than distance, conflict. (Wangh, in a personal communication, 1979). Inherent in this view is the assumption that conflict can never be truly resolved but can only be mastered by distancing from it. Dance-movement therapists who have thought about this dilemma agree, up to a point. Much human conflict is dealt with by repressing some portion of it so that the individual can go on functioning (Freud, 1915; Schoop, 1971; Schmais, 1974; Siegel, 1973; 1979; Espenak, 1979). Many people appear to disavow the affect states associated with conflict. But what happens to these split-off components of life experience?

The psychoanalytic community believes that they reside in the unconscious. So do dance-movement therapists. But they add to it the assumption that the repressed and forgotten fragments of experience are also still stored in the body. This is in agreement with Freud's (1910) formulation that the mind is never independent of physical-chemical processes and that emotions as well as instinctual gratifications and frustrations do not consist of mere thought but of physical alterations (Fenichel, 1945). Many dance-movement therapists address themselves to the recovery of these components through motility in a dancelike form. Indeed, the vast majority of dance-movement therapists are skilled in doing so. Some, however, rather than using psychoanalytic interpretation, see their interpretive work as primarily directed toward meaning and images in movement to produce insight (Whitehouse, 1977; Dosamantes-Alperson, 1977; 1979). Two examples of psychoanalytic interpretation during dance-movement therapy follow.

***

Example 1[1]

Sandra had a diagnosis of "childhood schizophrenia." Sandra has been regressing and exhibiting increasing amounts of hallucinatory behavior. She retold a story of having gone to a mall and "picking Santa's nose till it bled." She was punished for this by not being allowed to eat her ice cream. Sandra would furiously pick her own nose, while saying "It's disgusting. I will hurt myself—make it bleed." She was often unable to dance or to do exercises during sessions.

The following interpretation followed as a result of knowledge of her past history:

Tx: Sandra, you are picking your nose.

Sandra: It's disgusting. Don't do it. It will bleed.

Tx: If your nose is running, I will get you a tissue.

Sandra: No tissue. (Other hand moves towards the inside of thigh.)

Tx: I think you would rather put your finger into your vagina.

Sandra: (Full attention and eye contact).

Tx: But you're afraid that you will hurt yourself and bleed.

Sandra: (Nose-picking stops.)

Tx: You will not hurt yourself or make yourself bleed by putting your finger into your vagina—all ladies bleed from their vaginas, once a month. It is called having your period. Girls get their periods when they become ladies. I bleed once a month also.

Sandra: (Still listening intently).

Tx: Sometimes, it feels good to put your finger into your vagina. It's not disgusting, but you *may not* do it in front of other people. You may only do it when you are alone—like in the bathroom or when you are in bed.

---

[1]Contributed by B. Blau, D.T.R.

Sandra: Like when I was a little girl.
Tx: Yes, like when you were a little girl, but when you
           were a little girl you did it in front of other people.
           You *may not* do that again. You may only do it when
           you are alone.
Sandra: (Smiling—remained reality-oriented and engaged in
           movement exercises during the remainder of our ses-
           sion).

Example II

Kristen is said to be autistic; she does not speak.
Kristen is a child who kicks and has difficulty fusing her aggressive and libidinal drives.

The following interpretation was made as a result of the
knowledge that Kristen had eye surgery during the state of
development when children are beginning to exert their
agressive drive in the service of independence, as a consequence
of being able to distance themselves spatially from their love object. The supposition was that, during the recuperative phase of
surgery, her hands were restrained.

Tx: Kristen, you are kicking and trying to hurt me.
Kristen: (Smiling—continues to kick).
Tx: You may be angry at me, but you may not kick me.
           Here—kick the ball.
Kristen: (Quick thrust at ball with feet).
Tx: You may stamp with your good, strong feet on the
           good, hard floor. You cannot hurt the floor.
Kristen: (Performs exercises involving stamping and pushing
           floor, with feet and legs, while seated between
           therapist's legs).
Tx: (Hugging Kristen). You tried to hurt me, but hug-
           ging is nicer. I will not hurt you. I will not hold down
           your hands so that thety cannot move, like when you
           were a little baby in the hospital.

Kristen: (Lies totally relaxed, accepting libidinal contact, against therapist's body).

These examples clearly illustrate that clarifying, reassuring, structuring and genetic aspects of interpretation were useful in providing an avenue for change in the feelings and action of the youngsters involved. It is noteworthy that none of them had been accessible to verbal intervention before dance-movement therapy interaction.

With people who are more evolved, the proportion between dance-movement therapy and interpretation is altered, but not the basic model of movement interactions and interpretation as mutually complementary. While many people understand what they are dancing and moving about right from the beginning of therapy, others maintain a split between body and mind that can be astonishing. For instance, Mrs. H was a social worker who was also a formidable athlete. While she blandly and correctly examined all her movement qualitites, improvised with alacrity upon a theme and interpreted her own dreams with deadly accuracy, she found it comfortable to deride the therapist for her lack of neutrality in being visible instead of sitting behind the couch. Eventually a "game" evolved in which the therapist was the analyst and Mrs. H was an analysand. With surprise she discovered that she was "frozen" in the analytic position, i.e., she could not associate at all in the supine position on the couch. This was used to demonstrate her resistance to the therapist and to pave the way for recognition of her splitting.

In this context, it was the split between body and mind, not splitting of the ego as the term is used in psychoanalysis. Mrs. H had to heal her particular split by alternating between the use of the analytic postion on the couch and dance-movement therapy. Most others recreate their life history in the studio in such a fashion that at first there is an improvement, followed by slow regression to the fixation point, the place in their lives where the conflict first arose. The goal is always to

keep the regression confined to the treatment room by interpretation so that the client knows what he or she is experiencing. During this time movement-interaction predominates.
Then, as new patterns of meaning and being and creating are
established, the verbal interactions supercede the movement activities. The end result of this recreation of life's cycle manifests
itself in the ascendancy of unconstricted but controlled motility
and speech under the domination of a flexible self. In the retrac-
ing of life histories, the healthy desomatization a child would
achieve when it learns to substitute thought for action is
regularly encountered. When clients reach this stage and still
wish to dance, they are provided with a list of dance studios
where they can try their artistic wings on their own.

THE CONFLICT-FREE EGO SPHERE

Another psychoanalytic idea of great importance is encom-
passed in psychoanalytic dance-movement therapy; the concept
of the "conflict-free ego sphere." (Hartmann, 1958). Hartmann coined this term in order to delineate "that ensemble of
functions which at any given time exert their influence outside
of the region of mental conflict"(p. 8). He concerned himself
with those areas of human development that shape adaptation
in a peaceful rather than a conflictual manner. He pointed to
the fact that it is much easier to see the difficulties that arise
when strong emotions complicate adaptation than that the same
emotions also play a role in problem-solving and mastery. For
instance, a college student may be so furious that his parents no
longer pay his tuition that his grades become poor. His anger
and disappointment have overwhelmed his intellectual functions temporarily. But underneath it all he is goal-oriented. He
eventually finds another source to fund his studies. One can
view this incident from the frame of reference that the young
man was overly dependent on his parents and therefore overwhelmed by resentment and anger when they refused to support his plans, or one can focus on the same incident and see

that his anger propelled him into solving his problem and perhaps helped him to become more independent. While he was angry and disappointed, his goal-orientation and problem-solving abilities, as well as his grasp on reality, remained sufficiently intact to pull him out of his resentful state.

This has important implication in therapy. Clients whose strengths are acknowledged trust the therapeutic process more readily and form a working alliance fast. This, in turn, allows them to inch toward their conflicted areas with a degree of confidence not available to someone who is aware of conflicts only.

For instance, a young man, Neil, came to therapy because he was so tense and anxious that he regularly aggravated his baseball teammates by hesitating too long when at bat, eagerly running into them when trying to reach bases, and screaming their victory slogan when they were losing. He had difficulty in all peer relationships and was at a loss to explain why he behaved so erratically when he consciously knew better. It wasn't hard to see that Neil was full of muscle tensions which increased at times of stress. He had trouble looking at the therapist and twisted and squirmed pitifully when relating his tale of woe. In this ''nobody-loves-me'' and ''I'm-too-dumb-to-change-it'' behavior a strong dramatic quality was noted. Neil knew how to make himself understood by choosing words eloquently, and accompanied them with large, sweeping arm movements which, admittedly, sometimes swept objects off shelves. Instead of zeroing in on his tight shoulder girdle, rocklike stance and uncontrolled use of space, he was encouraged to ''recite'' his complaints, i.e., he was asked for an exaggerated, theatrical presentation. He took great pleasure in this and soon switched to reciting poetry—Shakespeare's Sonnets, to be exact. As he relaxed he was asked if he felt like moving his body now while declaiming the verses of the Immortal Bard. Soon after that he emerged as an accomplished young actor who joined his school's drama club and was now ready to investigate the tight musculature and overwhelming anxiety that still prevented him from interacting fully with his peers.

With someone who was on a less evolved plane than Neil,

even better results were achieved with Hartmann's concept in mind. Tom, a young man of college age like Neil, was hospitalized. He went through life indifferently, with vacant eyes and a robotlike walk, an enigmatic grin on his handsome face. At first he was thought to be heavily medicated but this was not so. He didn't participate in his group movement sessions although he came to the studio when it was scheduled. He indicated "no" to the offer of individual sessions. He was particularly apt at picking up rhythms. When everybody else did their own confused version of rock and roll, or simply could not pick up the steady beat of a Polka or Mazurka, Tom was always tapping these rhythms on the windowsill or table. He was given drumsticks and was appointed "official drummer." He liked this so well that individual sessions became possible, where much time was spent in exploring various rhythmic patterns. Tom's passive rigidity melted as he began to drum his own accompaniment to recorded music or to conduct it. His ability to hear and to reproduce rhythms had remained unimpaired and offered the therapist a chance to contact him.

When going to "where the patient is" one needs to meet his strength (Blanck & Blanck, 1974, 1979). If he cannot acknowledge his own conflicted or resistant behavior at first, well, isn't making such conflict conscious the first order of business in therapy? Directly confronting someone with their inabilities will always reinforce resistance and produce anxiety. Entering gently through the open door of the conflict-free ego sphere alleviates additional upheaval for the clients even when that sphere has become only an isolated ego apparatus.

In perusing only some of these very basic terms and concepts of psychoanalysis it becomes apparent that ego psychoanalaytic theory is applicable in almost all phases of dance-movement therapy.

The following chart elucidates and ties together some more psychoanalytic concepts useful in the application of dance-movement therapy.

DEVELOPMENT OUTLINE AT BIRTH

All innate givens are present. Conscious and Unconscious are not delineated. From an UNDIFFERENTIATED MATRIX, id and ego must form.

THE ID

Contains the drives, LIBIDO and AGGRESSION.

THE EGO

Contains apparatus as of PRIMARY AUTONOMY. They are the precursors of perception, motility, intention, intelligence, thinking, speech and language. At first only pleasure and unpleasure are differentiated.

THE ORAL PHASE
All phases overlap and are mutually inclusive.
FIXATION POINT FOR AUTISM
THE NORMAL AUTISTIC PHASE — BIRTH TO EIGHT WEEKS

	Normal Motility	Process of Internalization	Drive Differentiation	Defenses	Level of Anxiety
Object Relations					
Interpersonal relationships. Neonate is unaware of mother and surroundings.	Waving of arms and legs. Random touching of body. Lifting head. Primary concern with proprioceptive and enteroceptive stimuli. Focus on internal rhythms. Tonic-neck-reflex. Rolls partway to side. Clenches fist	(taking in from outside) Self and object representations are merged.	Aggressive and libidinal drives are fused and often discharged inward.	Primarily somatic overflow and discharge reactions to preserve homeostasis.	Catastrophic due to immature perception.

(continued)

41

Object Relations	Normal Motility	Process of Internalization	Drive Differentiation	Defenses	Level of Anxiety
	around rattle, drops it. Makes crawling and kneeling movements when on abdomen. Sucks, and mouths and drools. At 3-4 weeks, shift to sensory-perceptive organs.				
Superego	Symptomatic Motility	Symptomatic Object Relations	Symptomatic Drive Differentiation		Symptomatic Defenses
Not yet present.	Awareness and total response to proprioceptive stimuli. Unmotivated random movements of extremities. Focus on own internal rhythms. Sometimes hyperactive, head banging, rocking, whirling, biting, self-stimulating behavior. Arches away and stiffens when held, squirms or is limp and placid. Overly sensitive or impervious to sensory stimuli. Movements are jerky, jumpy and disconnected. Little awareness of time and space. Shallow and arhythmic breathing.	Self and others including things, are merged. Eye contact is often absent, inside and outside are confused as are animate and inanimate. May bump into things and people.	Libido and aggression are present. Swings between them are frequent and unpredictable.		Overflow and discharge, but in higher functioning autist also. Introjection, projection, denial.

THE ORAL INCORPORATIVE PHASE
FIXATION POINT FOR SCHIZOPHRENIA
NORMAL SYMBIOSIS—EIGHT WEEKS TO FIVE MONTHS

Object Relations	Normal Motility	Process of Internalization	Drive Differentiation	Defenses	Level of Anxiety
Need gratification. (Mother is seen as feeder or breast, a part object.)	Holds up head, rolls over, can reach, clutch and scratch. When pulled to sit, there is no head lag. Head and spine are integrated.	Self and object are felt to be one unit, but a unit of two, *not* total merger. "Hatching" occurs at end of phase.	Slow separation of libido and aggression under dominance of libido (baby sucks thumb instead of biting himself). Primary narcissism.	Introjection, denial.	Fear of loss of significant person.

(continued)

43

Superego	Symptomatic Motility	Symptomatic Object Relations	Symptomatic Drive Differentiation	Symptomatic Defenses
Archaic precursor.	Hyperactivity or catatohia. Body distortions with and without fantasy content. Bizarre gestures. Head rolling. Rocking. Fusion of hips and torso. Fusion of head, neck and torso. Toe walking. Tension around mouth and neck. Drooling. Biting. Dystonia. Little or no awareness of time and space. Arhythmicity of breathing and speech. Ability at height of symbiosis to imitate others' rhythms totally. Hypotonia, locked joints, inability to recognize others' bodies, loss of inner body sensitivities, and heightened awareness.	Significant others are felt to be part of the self. The need to be gratified predominates with little awareness of others' needs.	Drives are differentiated but either libido or aggression may predominate and alternate to their extremes.	Introjection, projection, denial. Turning against the self. Fear of re-merging with object.

THE SEPARATION—INDIVIDUATION PHASE

FIXATION POINT FOR BORDERLINE PERSONALITY ORGANIZATION

RAPROCHEMENT: FOURTEEN MONTHS TO TWENTY-FOUR MONTHS

Differentiation: 5 to 9 Months; Practicing Subphase: 9 to 14 Months

Object Relations	Normal Motility	Process of Internalization	Drive Differentiation	Defenses	Level of Anxiety
Dependence on mother decreases demarcation of self from her takes place. Ability to leave mother to explore environment.	Sitting, crawling, awareness of space. Standing, stretching up on toes. Playing peek-a-boo. Waving, touching of body, walking, lifting and replacing feet in same place, feeds self, can lean forward and stand erect, grasp pellets, waves and shakes objects, removes and piles up objects.	Mother is seen as separate but kept close. She is visually and tactilely explored. A primitive, but distinct body image occurs. Object constancy begins. Differentiation between self and others begins and slowly firms up. Ambitendency may exist.	Libido begins to tame aggression, but sometimes aggression overwhelms and temper tantrums result.	Splitting, undoing, regressions.	Fear of loss of significant person and of the self. Maybe free floating.

(continued)

Superego	Symptomatic Motility	Symptomatic Object Relations	Symptomatic Drive Differentiation	Symptomatic Defenses
Identification with the progressor via identification with the mother who gently weaned the child. The first prohibition against an instinctual wish can take place.	Vascillation between ability to do everything or nothing, erratic body rhythms, unclear use of space, misidentifications of inner body sensitivities, swings between good and poor performances. Shallow breathing patterns, occasional hyperventilation.	Intense swings between idealizing and devouring significant others. Inability to tolerate frustration of omnipotent or narcissistic wishes.	Intensification of aggression in relationship to introjection of "bad" objects.	Splitting predominates here as in other areas. Fear of and wish for remerger with significant others is also present.

THE ANAL PHASE
FIXATION POINT FOR OBSESSION COMPULSION
ANAL AGGRESSIVE AND/OR ANAL RETENTIVE 14 MONTHS TO 3½ YEARS

Object Relations	Normal Motility	Process of Internalization	Drive Differentiation	Defenses	Level of Anxiety
Weaning and toilet training becomes possible because mother is beginning to be seen as a separate person.	Walking, running, hopping, grabbing (spine is still held too rigidly for constant support. Abdomen is thrust forward. Weight on thighs, not centered above feet). Around 24 months can walk up and down stairs, at 36 months alternates feet. Jumps down from stair. Rides on tricycle, can stand on one foot, builds tower of blocks, unbuttons, traces, puts on shoes, etc.	Self and others are clearly delineated. An object and self representation exists internally.	Some frustration tolerance exists, neutralization of both drives is taking place due to gratifying and frustrating contact with a constant object. Discharge can be postponed. Ambivalence. Anal erotism.	Isolation, reaction formation (shame disgust). Undoing intellectualization.	Fear of castration.

(continued)

Superego	Symptomatic Motility	Symptomatic Object Relations	Symptomatic Drive Differentiation	Symptomatic Defenses
Reaction formation to please the mother allows for toilet training.	General body tension, particularly around sphincter and buttocks. Erotization of anus. Erect, rigid posture. Tight neck and shoulders. Inability to swing pelvis. Flattened feet. Strong but constrained quality in all movements or the opposite of all the above. Excessive sloppiness. Stubborn. Slackness of all muscles. Highly structured and constricted use of rhythms. Denial of body feelings. Hypochondriasis. Inability to read body signals correctly. Shallow breathing pattern with fixed rhythms.	Heightened ambivalence, defiance, rage and masochistic tendencies. Sometimes promiscuity.	Markedly aggressive or passive aggressive, marked anal erotism. Impotence or frigidity.	Excessive guilt or disavowal of responsibility. Rationalization.

THE PHALLIC PHASE
FIXATION POINT FOR HYSTERIA
THREE-AND-ONE-HALF TO SIX YEARS

Object Relations	Normal Motility	Process of Internalization	Drive Differentiation	Defenses	Level of Anxiety
Object constancy (an object can be loved despite frustration and disappointments).	All gross and fine motor patterns can be achieved. At 4 yrs. hopping on one foot, broad jump, throws overhand, laces shoes, builds buildings with blocks, dresses and undresses. At 6 years skips using feet alternately, jumps and lands on toes, catching own weight, body image is completed.	Identity and sense of self emerge.	Oedipal (libido is directed to parent of same sex at end of phase. Masturbation and urethral erotism. Sublimation becomes possible.	Repression	Fear of superego. Anxiety becomes a signal only.

(continued)

Superego	Symptomatic Motility	Symptomatic Object Relations	Symptomatic Drive Differentiation	Symptomatic Defenses
Identification with the aggressor (mother and father are right) including the ability to say "no" involving the use of aggressive drive in the service of identity.	Diffuse gestures. Directionless, but profuse motility. Restricted pelvic swing. True conversion symptoms with fantasy material. Partial anesthesias. Partial paralysis. Fusion of sensory modalities. Cramps, headaches, confusion of directions. Poor placement in both time and space. Vacillation between arhymicity and total recall of rhythmic patterns of others. Shallow breathing patterns.	Exaggerated indifference or adulation, emotive but shallow affect. Promiscuity.	Deeply repressed, little access to unconscious.	Overt urethral eroticism. Excessive preoccupation with masturbation or total denial of sexuality. Frigidity or impotence.

LATENCY

7 to 11 years: Libidinal Drives temporarily abate.

PUBERTY

11 to 14 years: An oedipal resolution is found with the help of all maturational and developmental levels.

GENITALITY

14 years to maturity and throughout life: The biological capacity to achieve orgasm is complimented by the ability to love another nonnarcissistically, to achieve intimacy and the ability to regress in the service of the ego. The establishment of a cohesive internal structure with an ego that is flexible enough to cope with id and superego demands.

This chart is based on the research of
Brown and Menninger (1940), **R. Fliess** (1948).
and **R. & G. Blanck** (1968, 1974, 1979).

Chapter 2

TOWARD A COHERENT THEORETICAL STRUCTURE FOR DANCE-MOVEMENT THERAPY

In the kind of dance-movement therapy proposed here motility is viewed an indicator of developmental levels, as an expressor of internal conflicts, and as a receptor that is imprinted with the reactions to all past and present experiences. Given all these properties along with the fact that it can be influenced, motility is a tool for therapeutic intervention. It can be another "ego apparatus" like speech, although not as specific. Both speech and motility are necessary to convey a complete message. This is true for both therapist and client. But while the client has the freedom to relax into "whatever comes up," the therapist has to fit into the context provided by the client's life experience.

MOTILITY ITSELF

The concept "motility" here encompasses not only functional motor skills, but all "motion" behavior of either a volitional or nonvolitional nature. Included in the moving behavior are its counterparts, States of Stillness. Thus, motility encompasses both Active Moving that is either consciously directed or not, and States of Stillness which, in a similar fashion, may or may not be consciously directed.

Active Moving and States of Stillness which are consciously directed are presumed to express varying states of perceptual awareness, triggered by stimuli from within and without. Perceptions coming from within include observations of thought processes, affective states, and bodily sensations, while those coming from the outside might be responses to any of the myriad stimuli impinging on the human organism.

For the present perception is seen as one of the essential functions of the mental apparatus which translates sensation into psychological representation. One can feel something on the sensory level but not acknowledge it, or have no tool with which to acknowledge it. Therefore, sensation precedes perception. Consciousness, on the other hand, includes perception and the ability to direct attention with intent to a given task, goal, or person. All these factors also connect with Motility.

To be complete, Motility must include yet another element: Intent. Intent can be roughly translated as a goal direction toward persons, things, or tasks.

Conscious, Active, Intentional Moving and Staying Still may also be freely associated as in "improvisation." However, the ability to move freely from one mode or level of complete motility to another is the is the outcome, not the process of psychoanalytic dance movement therapy.

Any given session will prove that clients earnestly strive not to hold anything back but are still barred from access to their own issues. They literally "freeze" themselves into a state of noncommunication that nevertheless is communicative in its mode.

Of course, Motility in and of itself is merely one of the many ways in which people express themselves. It seems to be, however, the only way in which a person can exist totally, without a body-mind dichotomy: i.e., one can simultaneously move and verbalize, choosing many modes of expression. As Schilder (1950) determines, "every sensation has its motility . . . sensation has in itself a motor answer. Continued activity is therefore at the basis of our bodily selves" (p.105).

Using motility in all its facets eradicates the age-old split between the body and the mind. The Cartesian view of the body as a machine directed by the mind, the presumed superiority of the "soul" which inhibits the hollow shell of an inferior body, comes to grief as frame of reference when confronted with motility. We live in, with, and through our bodies, and Motility remains unavoidable as long as we are alive.

EVOLVED MOTILITY

Conscious, Active, Intentional Moving and Staying Still in all its aspects is the most evolved form of motility. It can manifest itself in either so simple and ubiquitous an action as a firm handshake, or one as complex as a fully choreographed dance. It is not the form or complexity of motility that indicates its most evolved state but the clarity of its intent.

Clarity of intent can be achieved only when there is a mimimum of conflict. A limp wrist, for instance, can convey to the recipient of a supposedly welcoming handshake that he is not so very welcome, while lack of cohesion in choreography may leave the audience puzzled or bored. (Excluded here are those dances that are meant to puzzle).

Clarity of intent is present at all developmental levels and thus constitutes the major component of Evolved Motility. A toddler's firm and joyful pursuit of a ball encompasses for him all the above-mentioned aspects of Evolved Motility despite the fact that the child's uprightness is still precarious. Each human developmental phase carries with it specific and recognizable properties which are built into the phase superceding it. Thus, evolved motility also conveys the phase-specificity of Spitz (1965). He postulated the existence of organizers of the psyche which are said to influence subsequent development.

When consolidation of these organizers does not occur, the psychic system remains inchoate and less differentiated.

Maturation proceeds nevertheless but imbalance results despite the plasticity of the infantile psyche.

An examination of Spitz' three organizers shows that they all carry with them a form of motility and intent. The first is smiling, which is a response that marks a new phase in the neonate's life; volitional perceiving, recognizing, and responding to a significant other via controlled motor-function. The second is the "eight months' anxiety" in which the child will not accept a stranger in place of the mother. Here, the sensory apparatus is already sufficiently advanced to achieve a relatively complex form of Evolved Motility: groups of skeletal muscles can be used in the service of directed action sequences, as in pulling away. The child is also able to adjust posture and equilibrium to express its wishes. The third organizer is locomotion. It should be mentioned here that the establishment of locomotion has a strong impact on interpersonal relationships and thus becomes the point at which one can speak of Evolved Motility as becoming completely available. Before that, one could logically speak only of incomplete though Evolved Motility.

In other words, neonates who smile as their needs are gratified by an important other outside of themselves, or manage to suck their thumb in order to gratify themselves, use the type of Evolved Motility available to them at this time of life. What is important here is to note the fact that Evolved Motility in either its complete or its incomplete form is not available to all people all the time.

MOTILITY AS A SEPARATE DRIVE

Unavailability has to do with repression, developmental levels attained, and with the strength of a particular person's motor drive. Mittelman (1954) postulates the existence of a motor "urge" similar to that of the oral, execretory, and genital ones. Following Freud's definition, he delineates the motor urge as a drive or instinct. An urge, in order to be recognizable as one, has to be connected with indentifiable body organs that carry out or are the source of an activity which has the quality of urgency. When discharge occurs, it leads to pleasure and satisfaction. Certainly all these components are present in the human motor urge. Mittelman chose the word "urge" rather than drive or instinct because there are certain pitfalls connected with them. Freud used the word *Trieb* for which no adequate translation exists. It has been translated as "drive" or "instinct." However, "instinct" conveys the idea that it represents an inherited and unchangeable pattern. But *Trieb* does not imply any such unchangeability. *Triebe* can be, and are, changed by influences from the environment. Freud even thought (1915) that they originated under the influence of the surroundings. Thus, when Mittelman sought to name this quality which he observed in connection with motility, he called it an "urge" although it has all the hallmarks of what is commonly called an instinct or drive.

Motility itself, then, can be the visible representation of a universal human drive.

Observations of many clients over a period of nearly 20 years have led this writer to believe that there is indeed a separate motor drive which manifests itself in varying degrees among people. All my clients appear to have a stronger than average motor drive for which they seek an avenue of expression. The amount of discharge that goes along with speech in verbal psychotherapy is simply not enough for them. Their need to move obstructs the insight otherwise gained, or prolongs investigations when there is no place for anxieties and strong affect states to vent themselves in a motoric way. Many of these clients are by no means more than expectably narcissistic, exhibitionistic, or unable to form a transference neurosis. The factor that appears to set them apart from their peers in verbal psychotherapy is the need to use their bodies more fully. Among psychotics and Borderline Personalities this greater need may well have to do with their earlier developmental fixation points. But in some people who meet all the criteria for what is usually called "analyzability" (the ability to form strong transferences and to report in speech about inner happenings) there may still be an urge toward other forms of expression which has all the earmarks of a drive, and is in these instances a motor drive.

Freud (1915) had no objection to naming the existence of any number of drives, such as the drive to play, to destroy, or to be gregarious. He did warn that it might be more appropriate to look for the underlying components in these drives and to see if they could not be brought in line with the *Ur-Triebe* (primal drives), libido and agression.

In the case of the motor drive, I believe it to exist independently beneath libido and aggression because it can be used in coalition with either. In fact, I am tempted to postulate a motor drive as the only *Ur-Trieb* because no human situation can be without Motility, although in many individuals it has been so thoroughly tamed that it needs only minute escape hatches.

Freud speaks of drive stimulus *(Triebreiz)* which originates within the body and can only be satisfied by appropriate action. In his view, these drive stimuli act like a single push toward completion in action. He sees the prototype of action as flight from stimuli, whether as actually running from danger or as falling asleep in withdrawal. The drives themselves, however, are seen like a constant power *(konstante Kraft)* exerting their influences on both the somatic and psychic equipment of the person. Drive, then, straddles the physiologic and the psychologic. Flight is useless against the power of the drives because they originate within. One needs to find a way to satisfy them. Freud also delineates certain properties of drives: Their urgency *(Drang)* which represents their motoric momentum toward discharge; their goal of reaching satisfaction through extinction of the drive stimulus; the object through which, or on which, the drive can reach its goals; and their origins. Freud understood the origin of drive to be the somatic process in an organ or body part for which drive representation has been achieved within the psychic life through stimulus.

> . . . *jenen somatischen Vorgang in einem Organ oder Körperteil, dessen Reiz im Seelenleben durch die Triebe repräsentiert ist (p. 86).*

All these properties certainly are applicable to Motility, which regularly, and in all people, carries a momentum, has a goal, can attach itself to an object, and has its origins in the inner life of humans.

The urge toward discharge is stronger in some people than in others. Their need to be motorically active has not been tampered with by the demands of reality, or they have found a socially acceptable way of channeling their drive. This process must have taken place for them in the manner outlined by Freud in *Beyond the Pleasure Principle* (1920). He categorically links displeasure with an increase and pleasure with a decrease in the quantity of excitation. Thus, discharge takes on primary importance. Discharge, however, must always be linked up with the muscular apparatus and thus in some way with Motility.

The fact that the reality principle must supersede the pleasure principle is determined by the need to survive. Many clients give up their strong motor drive in order to live peacefully within the demands life places on them. When the restrictions are lifted in dance-movement therapy, they joyfully throw themselves into much motor activity once more. In other individuals this process is less clearly visible but still present. When the pressures toward conforming are too strong, there is nothing for the motor drive to do but to go underground and to seek another avenue of expression, even though what is consciously felt after this process is displeasure. Freud (1920) maintains that "all neurotic displeasure is in essence pleasure which cannot be felt as such."

> . . . *aber sicherlich ist alle neurotische Unlust von solcher Art, ist Lust, die nicht als solche empfunden werden kann (p. 22).*

In many instances, Freud's word *Unlust* has been translated as anxiety or even pain (Jacobson, 1953). This has grave implications for treatment because certainly therapists' responses would vary depending on whether their client were experiencing anxiety, displeasure, or pain. In an earlier (1905) treatise, Freud links the feelings of pleasure with muscle activity and even speculates whether pleasure is aroused through the perception of passive movement which is sexual in nature or whether it (the movement) is sexually arousing. In this statement, Freud also seems to be struggling with what comes first: Motility or another drive that lent Motility its quality. Children are assigned the permission for satisfaction of active muscle use *(aktive Muskelbetätigung)* and the question is asked secondarily if this safisfaction of muscle action might also have a component of sexual gratification. This same question is still asked today by those people who fear that the use of movement and muscle activity might be too gratifying and, thus, dangerous.

Actually, Motility itself is neither libidinous nor aggressive until other drives merge with it. One can reach out toward other persons libidinously and stroke them gently, or reach out and box their ears. In either example, the motor act and motor drive reaching-out existed before the other drive that gave it urgency and a goal. This is further evidence that Motility could be the *Ur-Trieb*.

It has been mentioned that there are people who appear to have a stronger than average motor drive and that they are the ones who find their way into dance-movement therapy along with others whose mastery of motility is inadequate. There is also a third, and perhaps larger group who are content without using their bodies vigorously. This does not have to do only with the desomatization that occurs during maturation and development. Rather, it is a statement about the fate of motility during life's vicissitudes.

Freud thought that drives can be diverted or used in many ways. He saw that they can turn into their opposite, as love turns to hate when it is frustrated. Drives can also turn against the self as sadism which becomes masochism. Repression becomes an avoidance of unpleasure so that the original drive disappears from the surface altogether. Or sublimation occurs in which the original drive achieves expression that satisfies all internal demands of the person on all levels.

The parallel to Motility is again readily drawn. Motility in many people has become an acceptance of stillness and curtailment of motion, or the opposite of its original form. Motility as a self-punishing device can be observed among some athletes, dancers, joggers, and whoever else is invested in using their bodies masochistically as a machine only. The need to move can be deeply repressed and curtail creativity, or it can emerge in joyful, free activity as sublimation. Drives turning into their opposite or repression, can also have defensive and adaptive connotations. I see concrete examples of all these faces of the motor drive daily in my practice. The many versions of motor stillness run the gamut from catatonia to simple refusal to move.

Christopher comes to mind. He was a man in his thirties who lived with his mother and thought of himself as saintly. He was suddenly overcome by inertia that neither he nor his doctor could explain. Because he saw himself as an exemplary son who was merely looking for the "right woman" before he could marry, and who held a responsible job as a civil servant, he did not think of himself as someone who needed psychotherapy. However, as his inertia deepened, he thought it might be good to look for an activity which would not be "rough" like sports of any sort and which would not require him to consort with the "wrong sort of woman" as could happen during social dancing. In a conference between his doctor, his mother, and himself it was decided that he was to take up movement therapy.

The snail-like quality of Christopher's movements was not enhanced by his inability to pick up a rhythm or by his stubborn refusal to try anything new. He decided that he would come for three sessions to "unburden" himself. To his surprise, he found that he had absolutely nothing to complain about. According to himself he lived in the best of all possible worlds, abiding by the principles set forth by his religion. His only complaint was the horrible fatigue that beset him and for which no organic cause could be found. Strangely, he still felt this need to "unburden" himself. As he became more and more puzzled by his need to put down a burden he could not identify, his fatigue deepened and he started to go to bed immediately after work. He dragged into his sessions week after week, forced himself to do some callisthenics he devised himself, and finally decided that his therapist was quite ineffectual. When asked why he thought so, he was immediately overcome with confusion, manifested in blushing, rapid breath and a slight tremor throughout his body, and said he would pray not to have such thoughts again.

During the next session, it was suggested that perhaps one of his burdens was to be stuck with an ineffectual therapist. This time, meek Christopher heaved a sigh of regret and announced that although he really disliked his therapist intensely, he thought he was "stuck" with her because she already knew so much about him that it would be too inefficient and time-consuming, not to say tiring, to start with someone else. This tirade, the longest in the interaction so far was accompanied by large, sweeping gestures and the body tremor. As transferential difficulties were worked through, Christopher became less and less saintly and more and more accusative. His permission to mirror his movements was obtained. He thought he was being mocked when mirrored. This made him so angry that he forgot all caution, shook his fist, shouted, strode up and down the room, finally took a deep breath and announced that he would never return.

From this agonizing beginning, Christopher became an almost manic mover. He enjoyed his anger so much that he began to look for reasons to be angry at the therapist and always accompanied his denunciations with forceful pantomime. Concomitantly, he enrolled in a gym class at his job, took up volleyball and joined a hiking club. As his muscles gained new firmness and he began to be able to gauge his capacity for movement, his inertia disappeared along with his "saintliness." Much of his motor drive had been so tightly held in check that there had been little energy left for anything else.

Obviously, he was a very angry man who had chosen to bind himself into inactivity because his deeply religious mother had wanted him to be a priest in order to save him from the evils of the world. Christopher, however, wanted to be an athlete and, as a child, worked out whenever he could. Shortly after his father died, his mother caught him climbing a tree. Shocked, he fell down and broke both his legs. He took this to be a direct sign from heaven that he was to be punished for disobeying his mother who was alone in the world and needed him. He gave up his secret sports activities and devoted himself to becoming ''saintly'' with the results dicussed here. This fragment of a case history shows a good example of the motor drive turning into its opposite, as well as against the self in a massochistic way in which pleasure became displeasure and rose to the surface as inertia.

MOTILITY AS AN EGO APPARATUS

In the chart preceding this chapter it is shown that the ego evolves out of an undifferentiated state in which all properties of the new human being are already present. At first, instead of a fully formed ego there are many ego apparati present in their unevolved form. Some of them are assigned primary autonomy, i.e., it is assured that they are relatively safe from the encroachment of the drives. Among these ego apparati are perception, motility, intention, intelligence, thinking, speech, and language and the five senses. Freud saw the Ego as the master of motility, or, rather, the total self, in this case, motility. He says in *The Unconscious* (1915) . . . while the conscious possesses firm mastery of arbitrary motility and regularly withstands the onslaught of Neuroses only breaking down in Psychosis. . .

   . . . *Wärend die Herrschaft des Bewussten über die willkürliche Motilität fest gegründet ist, dem Ansturm der Neurose regelmässig widersteht und erst in der Psychose zusammenbricht . . .(p. 138).*

Observation of any given dance-movement therapy session with neurotic clients belies this assumption. The hold of the Ego and consciousness on motility is by no means so firm as Freud thought. People regularly are out of control of simple stretches and bends. Much squealing and shuffling and groaning accompanies squatting down on the floor. Sitting Indian-style is a veritable torture for many. While these movements perhaps do not quite fit Freud's concept of *wilkürliche Motilität,* the act of walking certainly has become an automatic arbitrary function for most. The rigidities, inefficiencies, and unconnectedness of many people's gait are visible to anyone just going out into the street and watching.

There goes a woman with a stride too long for her legs. She reaches so far in each step that her upper body careens along on top of her legs like a sailboat on waves. There goes a man who minces as though his thighs were sewn together. Another smashes his heels into the ground with such force that a small shock-wave seems to travel through his body each time he takes a step. Yet another paces languidly on the balls of his feet, while his companion stalks staccato patterns on the pavement.

If a dance-movement therapist were to take any of these people into a simple retraining session that could teach them to walk more efficiently, she would encounter resistances of great magnitude. Not that all these people would consciously defy her. They simply wouldn't have enough control over their motility to comply. So once again I must digress from my parent theory and postulate that only parts of motility are controlled by the ego, that far from being an ego apparatus of primary autonomy it could more correctly be classified as an ego appartus of secondary autonomy. This merely means that it has been influenced by its own drive component but has become free of it and thus now functions relatively independently.

The idea of a basic motor drive has been postulated before. It should now be added that because it is so primary, a true *Ur-Trieb,* its presence at birth is more visible and clearly defined than aggression and libido, and that its emergence as a function is tied to the vicissitudes of any drive—it must attach itself to a body part in order to be visible.

In a singularly descriptive passage that is often awkwardly translated, Freud (1923) likened the Ego to a rider on a horse named *Id.* Rider Ego has to control Horse Id's power. Horse Id, however, is very powerful and can only be controlled by being guided to the place it already decided to reach. By joining it, Ego provides structure to the power of Id.

This idea fits closely into the metapsychologic framework for Motility. An hypothesis emerges that the basic motor drive arises through stimulation by tension within the body which seeks discharge. The motor drive finds its executor in motility. In other words, the drive constellation of the total concept "motility" has its base in the id, while the executive function of the drive are connected to motility itself in the service of the ego. Motility "rides" the motor drive. Both motor drive and motility are influenced by maturation, development, and the environment, and most specifically, in dance-movement therapy.

MOTILITY AS RECEPTOR OF LIFE'S EXPERIENCES

All people must submit to the gentling of their motor drive during growing up. One aspect of this gentling takes place after certain motor skills are learned. When they are performed daily, it is not necessary to think about them. They become automatic. "Automatization" here is used in Hartmann's (1938) sense. Many motor acts are performed without awareness of the intermediate steps leading to them. For instance, sitting rarely involves the conscious thought "I must bend my knees and make sure a chair is there." One merely sits. This automatization frees one for action that is simultaneous, outer- or inner-directed and aware. The lack of Automatization can lead to constriction through stillness while the individual ponders whether to sit or not, whether the chair is safe, whether indeed he or she can sit.

These action-inhibiting thoughts may be the outcome of organic disease and impairment, or the result of phobic and/or delusional states. On the other hand, the lifting of Automatization may produce a fresh approach to old problems and stimulate creative intelligence (Schmiedeberg, 1933). Automatization, then, can, but does not have to, contribute to constricted tamed motility. At first glance it may appear to be so adaptative a function that it cannot be separated from the total motility of the individual. So elemental a task as walking may be profoundly affected by the lifting of automatization. A person may over-reach steps or mince. Someone who over-reaches while walking must lunge and bend forward to maintain equilibrium. Walking truly upright with steps attuned to the length of the legs and the size of the body produces a different *Blickfeld,* a different "field of viewing," that allows for a wider range of cognitive experiences. Mincing, on the other hand, freezes posture and keeps motion localized in the legs and feet. Thus the way in which automatization is used affords a glance at the past in the form of motility. Even if an individual develops fully and freely, there is a "tendency to persistence in psychological function and development" (Sandler & Joffe, 1967). It is suggested that primitive modes of functioning do not disappear but stay active in the present under the cover of more complex adaptive behavior. This hypothesis gives credence to the widely held but as yet only empirically substantiated view of dance-movement therapy that there is a "Body Memory," i.e. that all experiences are stored in the body, specifically in the muscle systems, and are recoverable under appropriate circumstances.

A minute "dance" often occurs between partners in a conversation. As one leans forward to make a point, the other "closes up" by crossing legs or arms, or becomes "receptive" by shaping his body in complementary fashion. People who do not respond on this level are often considered less than affectionate by their peers. They are considered "haughty" or distant because their spines do not bend with the shifting winds of the surrounding conversation. Yet it would be erroneous to speak of a "conflict" here, certainly of an inner one, with such scant evidence. These individuals may indeed express a need to be distant, but their upright posture may instead merely reflect training and thus reproduce the ideals of their surroundings together with their own. If, however, there is a complete inability to relax such a spine there might indeed be something amiss. Conflict has created a constriction of motility over and above the expectable traces from the past.

Desomatization has been discussed earlier. In the present context this substitution of thought for action must also be mentioned as one of the factors which gentle the motor drive. If we followed all our motoric needs all of the time, an incredible whirlwind of motion would prevent us from stabilizing our actions at all. There is a distinct advantage in being able to think, "I could kill that guy," instead of committing the murder. The tragic consequences of an inability to control the motor drive is evident in hyperkinesis. These "perpetual motion" kids may suffer their symptom from a variety of causes. In dance-movement therapy, they find vast relief because their activities become structured segments of experience which they slowly learn to control instead of chaotically diminishing their ability to attend. Automatization and desomatization then can be seen to be constrictors of motility in the service of harmonious living, but also as imprinted with life's experiences.

So far, it has been discussed which factors are necessary to produce the kind of motility that is useful for living. It can be seen that motility and the motor drive are ubiquitous. But in order to live fully and with one's motor drive and motility geared to one's need, yet another factor is necessary, namely frustration tolerance.

Freud (1916, 1917) said that in order for adequate reality testing to take place, immediate drive gratification must be relinquished so that by postponing it, more adequate and complete gratification can be achieved later (Kris, 1958). Spitz (1965) enlarges on this when he says

> *"The capacity to suspend drive gratification, to tolerate a delay in the discharge of tension, to give up immediate and perhaps uncertain pleasure, in order to gain this certainty of later pleasure is an important step in the humanization of man. It made possible the progress from internal reception to external perception, from passive perception to motor discharge in the form of action, eventuating in active appropriate alteration of reality . . . . " (p. 172).*

Without frustration tolerance, life becomes an impulse-ridden drama full of discharge action that is frequently destructive to both things and people. It can show itself in the enraged destruction of a piece of furniture because it supposedly stood in the wrong place, or in the inability to attend to a piece of work until it is finished. The motility involved may be on the overt exertion level, as in the first example, or carry only the small physical energy drain of reading or writing.

The four components enumerated: Automatization, the Tendency to Persistence in Psychologic Functioning and Development, Desomatization, and Frustration Tolerance, shape the motor drive and motility as they evolve, and leave their imprint. The random movement of a baby towards its mouth soon becomes "automatic" sucking and feeding; we never really forget how it felt to be rocked by mother or how to skate and ride a bike as the Persistence theory suggests; we desomatize as maturation proceeds and, it is hoped, think instead of act when this is called for; we learn to wait until our efforts in whatever direction come to fruition. Each leaves its imprint either as fruitful constriction or body memory on the way we move.

The four influencers, however, have a common denominator without which they would not be able to exert their influence. This is Repression. During Automatization, the original thought process needed to carry out the motor act is repressed. In applying the Persistence Theory it becomes apparent that whole life sequences are repressed. Desomatization perhaps involves the least amount of repression although the process of trial action in thinking revolves around not doing, i.e. repression or diminution of one aspect of Motility. Frustration tolerance quite overtly involves repression of immediate discharge. During favorable development, this kind of repression is in the service of more harmonious living and does not impose an undue energy drain.

MOTILITY AS AN EXPRESSOR OF CONFLICT

Freud (1915) saw repression as the result of an inability to flee from drive stimuli within the self. It serves to keep something out of awareness. He states that in the case of drive, flight cannot accomplish anything. The self cannot escape from itself. Later, rejection based on judgment will be a good weapon against drive stimulus. Repression is a first step toward judgment, a good compromise between flight and judgment.

> *"Im Falle des Triebes kann die Flucht nichts nützen, denn das Ich kann sich nicht selbst entfliehen. Später einmal wird in der Urteilsverwerfung ein gutes Mittel gegen die Triebregung gefunden werden. Eine Vorstufe der Verurteilung, ein Mittelding zwischen Flucht and Verurteilung, ist die Verdrängung"* (p. 107).

In other words, Freud sees the hard-pressed human organism coming up with a solution that will allow it to exist without undue tension and without really giving up anything. Under the cover of repression, the forces of the drives proliferate and make their own connections. The Freudian maxim that repression really only interrupts the connection to consciousness and nothing else, may partially explain why so many people are uneasy when confronted with movement. Their motor drive has been deeply affected by repression so that anything motoric has become suspect. This is not surprising in a society where intellect is priced so highly that some children know their ABCs before they are toilet-trained and others can count before they understand that it is possible to ask for food to still hunger instead of crying. In both examples, body signals are not understood, or negated. But this cultural preference alone can hardly explain the depth of repression of the motor drive and motility present in clients who come for dance-movement therapy. They are not totally uninterested in their body selves, or ashamed of them. They simply do not know that their bodies are the medium for being alive.

Freud thought that drive representation develops more completely when it is not disturbed by consciousness. He says that it (the drive representation) ramifies luxuriously in the dark and finds forms of expression. When these are translated and used to confront the neurotic, they appear alien to him or her. But they also frighten the neurotic because they appear to reflect an extraordinarily dangerous strength of the drive.

> *"Sie, die Trieb-Repräsentanz, wuchert dann sozusagen im Dunkeln und findet extreme Ausdrucks Formen, welche, wenn sie dem Neurotiker übersetzt und vorgehalten werden, ihm nicht nur fremd erscheinen müssen. sondern ihn auch durch die Vorspiegelung einer ausserdordentlichen und gefährlichen Triebstärke schrecken"* (p. 110).

This state of affairs seems to be a regularly occurring event for the motor drive. Clients always claim that they cannot move, or, if they are willing to give it a try, find that they cannot do so freely. But when the repression is lifted, remarkable results are often obtained. Specifically, this means the freed motor drive which is connected with the observing functions of the ego. Before self-observation and self-awareness are brought into play, only catharsis can result when the motor drive is released. But when repression lets go of its strangehold, energy is freed. If this energy is motor energy, it will manifest itself in an increase of motor activities.

A case earlier cited is that of Christopher, who became a ballplayer, hiker, and gymnast all at once. There are many others who go to such extremes. There was Linda, who went camping and spent 18 hours of folk-dancing; and Pru who took dancing lessons, fencing, and aerobics all in one day. With others, the results are more modulated, but all seem to celebrate their new freedom with an enormous increase of motor activity. It is as though their motor drives while hidden under the shield of repression had gathered redoubled forces that must now see the light of day at all cost.

Constricted Motility then, is always an indicator of repression. But repression does not occur unless a conflict is also present. During maturation and development there are unavoidable conflicts in the service of meeting reality. Some of these also involve repression, as has been outlined before. But these do not create havoc. They smooth the way toward appropriate execution of motor functions. The deepest kind of constriction takes place when Motility—both the motor drive and motor functions—are forced by conflict and trauma to abrogate their vigor.

Fenichel (1945) describes the constricting situation well:

> *"The physical effects of the state of being dammed up emotionally are readily reflected in the muscular system. Pathogenic defenses generally aim at barring the warded-off impulses from motility . . . thus, pathogenic defense always means the blocking of certain movements. This inhibition of movement means a partial weakening of the voluntary mastery of movement"* (p. 246-247).

He further speaks of patients who have spasms which increase in intensity when their hidden conflicts come to the surface so that the spasm is a device for keeping emotional secrets locked away. He is also aware that

> *"muscular expression of an instinctual conflict is not always a hypertonic one. Hypotonic muscular attitudes, too, block or hinder muscular readiness . . . Dystonia and intensity of repression are not necessarily proportionate to each other"* (p. 98).

These statements could be a generalization of the symptoms many clients of dance-movement therapy show me. There was Doug, who thought of himself as a terrific disco dancer, but often had to limp from the scene of his triumphs because cramps hindered his dancing when he partnered young women. There was Eleanor, whose back stiffened into helpless rigidity every time her husband approached her sexually; Pam, whose clenched jaw ruined her teeth because she needed to hold in screams; little Petey whose luminous eyes never expressed the same spite as the vicious "involuntary" kicks he gave his mother—the list is too long to enumerate.

Another response to trauma is resomatization. During resomatization an adult ego is said to have misread the demands of certain drives as too dangerous. In its aim to eliminate danger, the ego refuses to allow these internal demands access to the motor apparatus and thus discharge. In evaluating the danger, the panic button was pressed by the ego as though it were about to be destroyed. In an instant, the whole maturational path is reversed. Thought as an "experimental dealing with small quantities of energy," (Freud, 1923) is lost and the individual slips into a global response to imagined internal danger. The end results of this process are the well-known group of psychosomatic diseases. But this is not the only way clients show constricted motility or motility as an expressor of conflict.

Examining the feeling states of my clients and how they deal with them by either denying their existence or adapting them to suit their purposes also affords me a view of constricted motility. The affective states are, in Freud's view, what is left over in consciousness of the original drives. Affective states all have their own specific motoric expression. It is not hard to see when another person is sad, or angry, or feels pain. Body posture, facial expression, and gestures express how the person feels. Some people are more "readable" than others, but all use their motoric equipment to signal to the world about their internal state of affairs. The English noun "affect" merely means "inward feeling on disposition" (Webster, 1949) but has come to carry other connotations in psychologic usage and particularly in psychoanalytic language.

In 1915 Freud stated that he thought a drive is either completely repressed so that none of it remains, or it appears as a somehow qualitatively colored affect, or it is transformed into fear ("anxiety" in the Standard Edition). The two latter possibilities confront us with the task of viewing the transformation of psychic drive energies into affect and especially of viewing fear (anxiety) as the new fate of the drives.

> "... Trieb, der entweder ganz unterdrückt ist, sodass, man nichts von ihm auffindet, oder er kommt als irgendwie qualitative gefärbtexe Affekt zum Vorschein, oder er wird in Angst verwandelt. Die beiden letzten Möglichkeiten stellen uns die Aufgabe, die Umsetzung der psychischen Energien der Triebe in Affekt . . . als neues Triebschiksa[1] ins Auge zu fassen" (p. 40).

Later (1926), Freud changed his opinion about the transformation of basic drive into fear, but the concept of affect as representative of the consciously perceived expression of the underlying instinctual process was retained. He also saw affect (1915) as manifesting itself "essentially in motor, secretory, circulatory changes in the subject's own body without reference to the outside world, motility in actions designed to effect changes in the world." He seems to have distinguished between affect and feeling, a Jacobson (1953) points out. The word "affect" seems to designate all psychophysiologic discharge phenomena. The physiologic components express themselves in body changes that are under the control of the vegetative nervous system. Examples are blushing, sweating, crying, increased peristalsis, rapid pulse, etc. The voluntary skeletomuscular system may be activated as well. Posture, facial expression, and tone of voice would be mediated by the peripheral nerves.

The psychologic components are experienced as "feelings." Rappaport (1950) sees affects in their psychosomatic

---

[1]*I have chosen to translate Angst as fear rather than as anxiety in order to clarify the qualitative difference. Earlier I spoke of the difficulties in translating "Unlust" as anxiety. Here, the same word, anxiety, has been used for Angst. The difference between Unlust and Angst is more closely approximated by using the English words displeasure and fear.

completeness and maintains that if there is no direct and momentary expression on either the physiologic or psychologic levels, ''a chronic alteration of the physiologic process as seen in psychosomatic disorders or of the psychologic process as seen in neuroses, psychosis, and character disorders may occur.'' However, as can be seen in looking at somatization in its various aspects, immediate or complete discharge of a given stimulus will not necessarily prevent the untoward events proposed by Rappaport. Rather, it is postulated that when one is forced by external or internal events to be adapt to life in a manner that is considered for that person, there might be something in those events that does not allow the individual to integrate, or ''digest,'' them sufficiently. Most often it is found that the person in question lacks ''frustration tolerance.'' So much of the original motor drive has been repressed that it now eagerly leaps to the surface whenever the smallest path opens itself. These exceptions are removed from their original aim due to repression. Lack of frustration tolerance is really a failure of appropriate repression.

This has important implications for therapeutic intervention because it becomes apparent that simple release of tension or abreaction may complete what the original stimulus, expressed in affect, had intended; but that the completion of it might stir up further conflict, being unmodulated and thus overwhelming. The affect must be released and completed in such a manner that the person feeling it can link it cognitively with appropriate mental representation and life experience so that closure and integration can take place.

It has been noted by Gestalt psychologists, in particular Zeigarnick (1927), that unfinished tasks are remembered, while finished ones are forgotten. Therefore when a child is told *no* he will recollect the experience easily because he could not carry out his intent. He has been frustrated. But if this affect, frustration, is brought about within a trustful relationship with a prohibitor, the mother, he will identify with her and begin saying *no* himself (A. Freud, 1936).

This simple identification with an ''old'' aggressor (an aggressor from the past) is often a component in affective states and must be taken into account. If only the release of affect is accomplished, the components which caused it may still be hidden and even receive exaggerated importance through their artificial isolation from the emotive part. Release in and of itself does not mean completion, as is outlined in the discussion of lack of frustration tolerance. If the person in question was not able to establish "frustration tolerance" as discussed above, a release of affect may bring about less of boundaries. So, before beginning the release and relaxation techniques known to any reasonably well-trained dance-movement therapist, it is essential to ask: What is the expected result of this affect is indeed completed in its entirety? What kind of new affect will appear in its place? And with what developmental level will the client come in to touch?

The answer must be that the muscular release has to be connected with the original thought and events—representation by careful linking of past and present. It is only when the past is mastered that we are free to be in the present. Overwhelming or inappropriate affect destroys the present.

Psychoanalysts have long viewed strong feelings with concern. In 1941 Fenichel spoke of affects as "archaic discharge syndromes" and of "affect spells." This thought is echoed by Krystall (1978) in his description of affect storms. They seem to imply that strong feelings ought to be tamed enough not to find motor expression. This idea is anathema to the kind of dance-movement therapy proposed here. Affect is so strong a link in bridging the inner and outer world and closes the gap between psyche and soma so completely that it is the most complete approach tool which can be found. Affects are concrete, visible, felt, lived, and transmittable agents of the body-mind unity. They must be brought into their most evolved form in order to become a vehicle both for discharge and self-observation. It is the incompleteness of affect that makes for trouble.

The client Merce comes to mind. She habitually used her hands in a groping fashion, never relaxing her fingers for one moment as she talked. Even when occupied in gross motor activities, she returned to her "groping" as soon as a sequence was ended. She could stop herself from this behavior, but reported that a pressure sensation would settle in her stomach if she desisted. Her verbal associations pointed in the direction of "being picked on in sibling rivalry," as she called it. These brought her no relief. It was also noteworthy that her associations were not connected with changes in rhythm of speech or breathing, as was usually the case for her when she was talking about significant events in her life.

It was suggested that she assume a supine position on the floor and consciously exaggerate the groping. While doing so, a light plucking motion came to light. However, nothing much changed in either Merce's feelings states nor in her associations. Sometimes the symptom would stop for a brief moment when I allowed Merce to hang on to my hand. Eventually, a dream revealed a painful fantasy about the loss of Merce's father, who in reality was alive and well. Merce's groping behavior increasing during the recital of the dream. She had long experienced her behavior as inappropriate, and had gone to some lengths to stop it. She now became aware of how frantically she was groping about. She rapidly reviewed, to no avail, her various theories as to why she couldn't stop herself. Her sudden pallor, rapid breath, and the ever increasing speed of her hands searching for an elusive something alerted me to the presence of intense feelings which stubbornly refused to be connected with content.

Finally, after torturing herself to be "good" and to "give associations," Merce commented that she felt she was wrestling, but did not know with what. She was given a long plush snake kept for just such "wrestling." Merce immediately began gleefully to wring its neck. She alternately stroked and fondled it, cooed to it, held it like a baby, and then again strove to pull it apart. Soon a happy three-year-old emerged who could play with the snake, put it to sleep, and sing to it. Then another fierce battle ensued in which the snake was ritually slain, and the session took on the turgid drama of the Grand Guignol. During this entire performance, Merce never once lost the ability to observe herself, and intermittently made mildly amused comments about her own behavior. She noticed that her hands were strong, that she could command rhythm in her actions and that there was something ridiculous in wanting to decapitate a plush snake.

It took several sessions to work through what had actually happened. Somewhat ashamedly, Merce admitted that she had always wanted to "tear her father limb from limb" after she had heard him shout at her mother. Her way of dealing with parental disagreement had been to run into her room and to play with her baby blanket, stroking it, tearing it, and hiding under it, depending on whether she needed a comforter, an opponent, or a safe place. She had acted then as she acted with the snake now. Later, she became a nail-biter who, in her own words, "bit her nails all the way down to her elbows." This anger at her father, along with an inability to form satisfactory relationships, as well as enormous amounts of free-floating anxiety, had driven her into treatment with a psychoanalyst. There, she insisted she had found no relief because she had to "lie still."

In contrast, in dance-movement therapy, Merce found a way to lift the repression which had bound her strong affect in incompleteness. Once the affect—anger—was connected with its goal and object—father—and its motility, we could set about examining the encroachment of the past upon her present.

Merce's strong need for motor discharge would have landed her in untoward "acting-out" without the opportunity to "act-in" during the sessions. Such acting-in is not overly gratifying. Rather, clients with strong motoric needs have shown that psychotherapeutic intervention would become a stalemate for them without opening the gateway to their own motility in their sessions. To date, there is no measure or assessment tool to determine who could best be served by psychoanalysis and who by psychoanalytically oriented dance-movement therapy. Self-selection and some developmental criteria so far delineate the population for dance-movement therapy.

It is assumed by many clinicians that only people who are stuck in the earlier developmental leves can benefit from dance-movement therapy. The body-image distortions, lack of appropriate motor behavior and need for tension discharge among autists and psychotics make them prime candidates. But the focus on Motility as both a drive and an ego apparatus widens the scope for the application of dance-movement therapy beyond these categories.

A brief discussion of development will show that the motor drive and motility are present in phase-specific form at all levels.

STAGE AND PHASES IN HUMAN DEVELOPMENT

The Oral Phase

The first stage for all human beings at birth is the oral one—an apt designation indeed. Anyone watching a baby in its first weeks of life cannot fail to notice that all things the little one encounters are related to the mouth. As soon as sticking the fingers into the mouth is recognized as something that brings gratification, everything else is brought into proximity with the mouth as well. Hoffer (1947) links these facts with the emergence of the first true body-ego; i.e., because there is a remembered state of pleasure in putting the hand or fingers into the mouth, the consolidation of an ego, or an awareness and directedness in action, take place.

In this directedness and awareness much is still missing. The baby acts as though all things could be eatable and bring pleasure, until it finds out otherwise. Just consider how many important discoveries can be made by putting the fingers into the mouth. Hard and soft become known in the exploration of bony gums and soft tongue. Warm and cold are more readily perceivable in that the finger taken out of the mouth cools off more rapidly than a wet diaper; thus the link between the two sensations can be made easily. The shapes of mouth, cheek, and chin can be traced and fingered and form the first perception of separate entities. This had led psychoanalysts to speculate that babies must first learn the difference between alive and not alive, inside and outside, self and not-self in a very laborious fashion. Everything is related to the mouth as the basic link between the world and the emerging self.

The beginning phase of life, the first 4 weeks or so, are called by Mahler (1968), the time of "normal autism." Everyone goes through this phase when even the rudimentary perceptions and sensations hinted at above are present only in fragmented and chaotic form. There simply isn't an organizing component developed enough for the neonate to use anything but tension discharge in order to feel good. The infant seems to be in its own shell, occasionally responding to physiologic discharge needs. The urge is first and foremost toward homeostasis. Autistic individuals never outgrow this state of affairs. They merely seem to settle more firmly into the rigidities and warding-off mechanisms of this very early time period.

Right after this "normal autistic," phase symbiosis between the mothering person and the baby takes place. The instinct for self-preservation is not so strongly developed in the human infant as in animals. The young human is dependent on its surrounding to a much greater degree and for a longer time. Some, including Freud, have speculated that a long dependence on parenting may in part be responsible for the development of neurosis. Being controlled and not being allowed to grow in self-gratifying ways could stir the cauldron of inner conflicts to unbearable levels. But the symbiotic phase is gratifying, and necessary for survival. The young infant needs the empathetic understanding of the mothering person in order to survive at all and in order literally to learn, through predictable, repetitious experiences, that tension and discomfort will come to an end eventually. Mahler (1975) describes succinctly how the infant at that time functions as though baby and mother were one overpoweringly strong unit. In this omnipotent relationship, the infant learns to differentiate the need-gratifier's face in connection with the appearance of tension release (Spitz, 1965). The baby is enabled to shift away from listening to predominantly visceral rumblings on the inside to predictable, and therefore safe occurence in the world outside. Concomitantly, the periphery of the infant's own body becomes a known entity to him through the ministrations of the mothering person.

In this shift from autism to symbiosis in normal development, an enormous variety of motor behavior has already evolved. At first, the baby rests in a supine position, the head usually to the side. Tonic-neck-reflex postures predominate. There is a headlag when the baby is pulled to a sitting position (Gesell, 1973). The baby may or may not roll to the side but when prone, and already tries to lift the head. He may make crawling movements, or wave its arms about like a swimmer. It often holds its hands in a fist and clenches articles put into its palm. While autistic adults and children often have learned how to walk, vestiges of this early time are visible in all their motoric behaviors. There is a wall of such extraordinary coldness between the autistic individual and the environment that the mothers of such people often report that even in early infancy they were unable to relax when held. The normal motility to be expected in the earliest time of life includes waving the arms and legs, random touching of the body, thumbsucking, drooling, and attempts to lift the head.

Symptomatic motility is characterized by arching, squirming, and stiffening or its opposite when body contact is made. (Some potentially autistic infants become limp or flaccid when held). There is also a marked sensitivity to sensory stimuli from both inner and outer sources. (Brody, Axelrad, Moroh, 1976). These stimuli are generally vigorously warded off both by diffuse discharge reactions or total withdrawl. Introjection (taking it all in) projection (spitting it all out), and withdrawal (it isn't there at all), are beginning to form as potential defenses. The levels of anxiety are overwhelming. Fear is never just being afraid. It is always of catastrophic proportions, because the fact that there might be help and nurturing in the world is forgotten or denied.

To lead the autist into a closer awareness of the self and others has been the privilege of many dance-movement therapists. In my own memory, special places are reserved for the first time Tommy tentatively touched my hair and stroked it. After many months of spotty interaction he finally decided it was okay to approach me this far. Hair, after all, still has an inanimate quality and can serve as a transition between touching and not-touching. Lida had no such qualms. She firmly grabbed my hand and used it to obtain a favorite toy. Jerry thought it would be nice to wear my shoes and became upset when he realized that they could be detached from me without my feet in them! Each in their own way laboriously recognized first only part of me as existing as an important Other outside of them. When full body contact could finally be established in a hug, we always had a special time with each other. But it was slowly that this spread to others, who also had to prove their trustworthiness first. Working with such adults and children is a continuous tug-of-war for me between when to intrude into those autistic shells and when to leave them alone. Most of the time, it is best to wait for a signal, as outlined above. But the autistic self is so fragmented it needs help to peek out. Therefore, one needs to watch for activity that can be joined and enlarged, i.e., I do not only "mirror," but ask both verbally and nonverbally: Try it my way!

Symbiosis

The schizophrenias are said to have their origin in the symbiotic phase when some part of that phase cannot be outgrown. (Fliess, 1948; Brown, 1949; Blanck, 1968; Rutter, 1979). A sociobiological unity between mother and child normally takes place in which the baby reacts in every way as though it and mother were one person who dominates the known world. The symbiosis is said to last from one to five months of age. Obviously the imprint upon motoric behavior here is great. Because all human agencies then are still both physiologic and psychologic, many infantile motor patterns are retained under more mature ones (Greenacre, 1958; Spitz, 1965). They resurface when a schizophrenic regression occurs.

By five or six months of age, many babies can sit and

begin to stand. They like to bounce, and can scratch, clutch, and rake things in with the palm. There is generally a good deal of motoric energy and initiative which is not merely repetitive. Enjoyment of all visual and motor explorations is fairly high and intentionally can be seen in gesturing and movements. The form and shape of a little person is already emerging and begins to tease the mind of the onlooker with speculations as to what sort of grownup this baby will become.

Similar vestiges and elusive ''almost'' phenomena pervade the motoric interactions in dance-movement therapy with schizophrenics. One needs to be alert to the low frustration tolerance and incapability for sustained emotional contact of these clients. Symptomatic motility includes hyperactivity and catatonia and all the gradations in between. Body distortions with and without fantasy content are regularly present. Bizarre gestures occur, as do head rolling, rocking, and grimacing. There is usually a fusion of hips and torso, or a fusion of neck, torso, and hip. Tensions around the mouth and neck are frequent, as are drooling, biting, and spitting. Rocking and toe walking are part of the usual movement repertoire. There is little or no awareness of time and space, and arhythmicity of speech and breath exist side by side. At the depths of such symbiotic regression, there is a total ability to imitate another's rhythms, but the imitation is forgotten immediately. Identification (I am like you) and displacement (No, I didn't do it; you did) are added to the defensive and adaptive strategies available. In illness, fear of being swallowed by the loved person is also present, so that all defenses are turned against the self. It's already a very complicated interaction!

In dance-movement therapy, the symbiotic client shows a way of clinging and exactly replicating movement that is astonishing. Jesse was one who could do absolutely everything in movement as long as his therapist was around but who shrank back into near catatonia and an ''institutional shuffle'' when alone. Together, we could dance a tango or a mazurka and discuss much of his life history, but no change occurred. One day, quite by accident, we bumped into each other so vigorously that we both fell to the floor. We had been doing our version of the "Bump". Jesse was amazed to note that his therapist didn't seem to hurt in the same place as he when we fell. He was then able to tell me that he assumed I went "into a black hole" when he had to return to his ward. The black hole represented the inside of his own head, as he told me the next session.

Jesse is very representative of other psychotic people I have worked with. They are damned if they do and damned if they don't: that is, if they allow the trusted person to become part of their inner world, they lose the person; if they, on the other hand, identify with the trusted one, they lose themselves, or so it seems to them. Adult or child, they need to define their body boundaries and often can only do so by touching another, and by being touched.

Separation-Individuation Means Becoming Oneself

The separation-individuation phase follows next. This phase is said still to belong to the oral stage, though anal factors are beginning to make themselves felt. Between five and nine months of age, the total bodily dependence of the baby on the mothering person begins to give way. As perceptual and cognitive functions mature, babies begin to differentiate from mother. They begin to explore mother's and their own bodies tactually and compare what they find to the world around them. Their own little body image expands from the first hand-mouth ego to include more of their own body. The term "body image" is meant to convey the felt, conscious knowledge of one's body (Schilder, 1950) as well as the inner representation of it. Mahler (1978) has called the differentiating process "hatching" and likens it to the psychological, rather than physical, birth of the human infant.

The development of locomotion comes into play as a major factor at about nine months. For the first time the baby is able to move away from mother or return to her, first by crawling, then by walking. How the members of the dyad handle this "practicing" period will leave strong imprints on all future behaviors. Along with the real ability to bite and chew, the wish to devour and to destroy also is present. Baby now can feel angry at mother, or have loving feelings toward her. It's really the baby's choice. But with tears in one's eyes or while caught up in an important game of exploration, it is sometimes difficult to recognize that it is one and the same mother who can make one so angry, or so happy. It takes "identification with the aggressor" (being like mother or any person who is in control) to bind some of that ambivalence arising out of the perceptual confusion. Some authors (Greenacre, 1958; Mahler, 1978) have linked pushing away from mother, or the refusal to look at her, or ignoring her comings and goings, as the precursor to the later psychologic defense of denial.

In dance-movement therapy at this stage, the adult or child needs encouragement to explore and dance by oneself, no matter how primitive this dance might be. Touching one another becomes much less frequent. If it is necessary at all, it is interpreted in order to maintain and shore up clients' autonomy. Their will toward finding gratification outside of treatment is nurtured instead.

The Anal Phase

At about nine months of age it becomes clear to young infants that they can expel something anally, or that they can retain it. The necessity to control the sphincter can become a battle fought too early or too late, or can take place naturally when baby wants to be "big" and make "big." But before that problem of growing up is solved, and overlapping the third phase in the struggle for separation and individuation, another important form of fixation can occur. Kernberg (1976) places the origin of the Borderline Personality Organization here. In the harsh vacillations between loving and hating one and the same person passionately, it seems as though the person suffering from Borderline Personality Organization like the toddler in the practicing phase, does not clearly recognize that he or she is dealing with one and the same person. Integration of hostile and loving feelings has not taken place, while many other ego functions have developed and reached maturer forms. These vacillations of feelings are also visible in the motor apparatus of the borderline patient in dance-movement therapy, who likewise is "practicing" running away from and coming to the therapist.

Rapprochement

From about fourteen months to two and a half years, the children are busy in the rapprochment stage. They find mother is neither part of themselves, nor an ogre, but a woman they need and love. This is a particularly difficult time, because without the omnipotent feelings of being merged with mother, or the equally powerful ones of wanting to destroy, now comes the realization that, far from being able to do anything, they are vulnerable. They begin to form reactions toward things they always accepted. For instance, the stool, instead of being a negotiable commodity with which to buy mother's approval or disapproval, now is found to be "disgusting," it smells bad. Shame and disgust begin to displace the more explosive reactions of babyhood. Small wonder, then, that this is also the time when temper tantrums, whining, and mood swings appear. It is fortunate indeed that by now, the child can run and hop and do all sorts of tricks in compensation for all that separating and following the dictates of reality!
Support isn't all that steady and needs the forward thrust of the abdomen for balance. Retaining and controlling are major activities. Reality demands are met more and more. Frustration tolerance is present and when fear is experienced, it is no longer of quite such overwhelming proportions. It has become "merely" the fear of losing a body part, or castration fear.

Obsession compulsion has its roots in this anal phase (Fenichel, 1945; Salzman, 1972). It is called anal because so much attention is paid by both child and environment to management of the sphincter muscle. Often, this includes great interest by both the parent and the child in the size, shape, color, and consistency of the child's stool. At the same time, however, as mentioned above, disgust and shame have been discovered. How to reconcile such interest with the newly acquired defenses? Easy. One learns to undo what one has done. (I didn't wet my pants. I washed them). One can also start telling tales and use one's intellect, as in intellectualization, or if need be, regress to earlier behavior.

Interestingly, many obsessive-compulsive individuals who do and undo, intellectualize and regress, also bring the toddler's stiff spine into dance-movement therapy. Quite often, there are general body tensions, particularly around the sphincter and the buttocks. The anus is perceived as an erotic aperture in reaction against the shame and disgust also felt. Posture very often is rigidly erect, with tight neck and shoulders. Flattened feet complete the picture, while the movement qualities are strong but constrained, or the opposite of all the above! Ambivalence is the key word describing the obsessive-compulsive patient.

In dance-movement therapy at this stage the adult or child needs encouragement to explore and move alone.

With clients who are fixated on this level the sessions look very different from those described earlier. The therapist hardly ever moves with them. After all, the search is for the clients' movement patterns. This search should not be contaminated by the therapists' more evolved and therefore more powerful movement patterns. A dance combination or a technique might be demonstrated but the emphasis is on *Do It By Yourself!*

The danger of producing emotional attachments that last too long is diminished in all phases of dance-movement therapy because clients are always encouraged to move and do it by themselves. This active doing counterbalances dependency needs.

***

The Phallic Phase

The next step on the developmental ladder, the phallic one, allows for the incorporation of genitals into the body image; but, just the same, some inner conflict rages around whether to masturbate or not. This conflict is said to arise whether there is parental prohibition or not. Boys begin to like their penis even more than previously, and girls their clitoris. Urinating becomes a fascinating activity. But, if all goes well, repression will take place, sublimation becomes possible, and the so-called latency period is ushered in. Should a smooth transition into the latency period be interrupted, hysteria is said to be the result (Fenichel, 1945; Krohn, 1978). It sometimes occurs that people with this diagnosis appear in the dance-movement therapy studio. One finds a lot of diffuse gesturing, profuse but directionless motility, restricted pelvic swing, conversion symptoms with and without fantasy material, partial anaesthesias, fusion of sensory modalities, cramps, headaches, poor placement in both time and space, as well as vacillations between arhythmicity and total recall of rhythmic patterns.

From there on in, puberty and true genitality with all its joys and pitfalls are ahead.

Puberty is a time of re-examination. Old answers can be expanded or discarded altogether. New constellations of interpersonal relationships may evolve. The entire range of past life history gets a going-over, as it were, so that both strengths and weaknesses in the personality have a chance to form the silhouette, at least, of the adult who will emerge. No insurmountable problems will come to the fore if all other stepping-stones in the oral, anal, and phallic phases have successfully been mastered. The young adult will stride into life with the confidence that the achievement of true genitality conveys. In this context, true genitality as a concept is not confined to the description of how one uses one's genitals. It is a shorthand employed to convey that a delicate but durable balance between psyche and soma has been reached that allows thought and action to function interdependently under the direction of a well-defined ego.

In summary: there have been discussed the many facets of Motility that must be taken into account if an in-depth, primary therapeutic intervention is to take place. No doubt there are other aspects that have not yet been conceptualized.

The important Latency Phase is not included because within the psychoanalytic framework it is not viewed as a time when fixations arise or the making of major neuroses take place. If something goes wrong during this period when all the drives are temporarily asleep, this is taken as a diagnostic sign that one or the other earlier developmental phases were already troubled (Freud, 1905; Blos, 1962).

The well-known fact that client and therapist must feel something about and for each other before any permanent changes can take place will be the focus of the next chapter.

Chapter 3

REACTIONS OF CLIENT AND THERAPIST TO THE CLINICAL RELATIONSHIP

The opinion is often voiced that technique and theoretical considerations in therapy do not matter, that what really counts is the quality of the interpersonal relationship between client and therapist. Overlooked in this opinion is the fact that the climate for such a relationship has to be created before it can surface. Further, psychoanalytic theory teaches that such a relationship tends to lead nowhere if the therapist does not recognize it and does not make use of what is transpiring. Willingness and intuition on the part of the therapist are simply not enough. An enthusiastic neophyte can even drive such a therapeutic relationship underground again, or can encourage it to lose all boundaries by superimposing her own feeling tones. A transference relationship becomes maximally useful to the client only if the therapist knows what to do with it.

In dance-movement therapy, a powerful element, Motility itself, creates a whole new dimension to transference that has not been examined in depth before. The notion that it is movement and motility pure and simple which effects changes for our clients reveals itself as romanticism. If moving and dancing were all that is needed one would merely have to go to a creative dance teacher and move about. What makes dance-movement therapy a vehicle for in-depth intervention is the fact that it can be employed to recover memories, to dissolve resistances, and to bring transferences to the surface. Experience has shown that some of these factors manifest themselves more readily and strongly in movement than in speech and therefore must be scrutinized with particular rigor.

Conscious, evolved motility enters the picture at a developmentally earlier point than speech. Therefore it is closer to the time when the psychobiological unity was more complete. Thus, when movement and motility are the primary mode for intervention, early memories are stirred up more readily than when they are approached through speech. Of necessity, the arousal of these early phenomena engenders stronger feeling currents than speech alone. These feeling currents must be channeled and structured quickly in order for them to be observed and integrated by client and therapist alike.

Because clients are "doing" and are in action while experiencing strong feelings, their excitation is channeled and structured by their own activity and self observation. This shores up body boundaries and body image, emphasizing the client's separateness. For instance, an anxious person who begins to gasp during breathing exercises may temporarily lose all sense of the here and now while reliving an early abandonment: as did Doris. Her tranferential need was to be held and to be rocked, something her mother had never done when she was hurt. Pointing out verbally that she was an adult now who could satisfy herself merely reinforced her need to be both dependent and angry. When dancing a waltz was suggested Doris found that she could gratify herself this way in the swaying and rocking that evolved out of the strong rhythmic flow of such music. Simultaneously she had another thought: suppose she asked her boyfriend to waltz with her? The two started social dance classes. Doris became able to look at her demands to be rocked by her therapist as a natural outgrowth of her early deprivations and at her simultaneous problem-solving as a step toward independence. The breathing exercises had evoked early memories and her need to cling. Moving by herself in a way that matched the early developmental need enabled her to "think" about her conflicts without being swamped by feelings.

Transferences are of such enormous importance in all forms of treatment, that they can be likened to the honey that traps the past and helps to construct a continuous path that leads to the present. Of course, the consistency of the honey varies! In symbiosis it can have the irksome quality of glueing everything together too sweetly, while during certain affect storms it yields no more adhesion than a little sugarwater. Without transference, clients lose the incentive for remaining in therapy no matter how brilliantly the movement interactions run. When it becomes too intensely positive or negative, treatment is interrupted prematurely or goes on interminably. Either way, the therapist needs to respond interpretively, in order to help the client resolve, not solidify, these emanations from the past.

Freud (1914) thought that transferences are an intermediate bridge between pathology and life. They allow the past to be recreated in the present. His idea was, of course, that the medium for the expression of such unconscious memories would be speech. In dance-movement therapy the expressive component for transference is most frequently Motility. But dance-movement therapy and psychoanalysis have this in common: they do not create transferences. They allow them to come to light and to develop in the fertile gound of the sessions, provided the therapists step out of the way long enough.

The American Psychoanalytic Association defines transference as "The displacement of patterns of feelings and behavior, originally experienced with significant figures of one's childhood, to individuals in one's current relationships. This unconscious process thus brings about a repetition, not consciously perceived, of attitudes, fantasies, and emotions of love, hate, anger, etc. Under many different circumstances . . . the types of transferences include intra - and extra-analytic situations, as well as positive and negative . . . potentially, it may develop between any two human beings''(p. 92-93).

In other words, no human interaction is free from the past, with that part of past experience that has been submerged in the unconscious constantly influencing perceptions and reactions in the present. That there is a dichotomy between fully experiencing the present and therefore responding freely to patient or friend while working from a given theoretical framework is strongly reinforced by the Existentialists, especially Sartre, who is convinced that the only authentic state of being-in-the-world is the noncommitted moment when all possibilities are open, when no possiblity kills off any other possibility.

Sartre also recognizes that this state of being-in-the-world can arouse profound anxiety since it is a preconscious rather than unconscious experience. The ego is already cognizant of the push toward action and the holding back causes conflict, hence anxiety. Any one action kills off the possibility of all other actions and is thus both absurd and inauthentic, according to Sartre's Existentialism. Since dance-movement therapists are in response to patients' needs, there would be a difficulty in using this framework to facilitate freedom from the past and integration of transference.

Intuiting all possibilities emanating from the clients could conceivably be achieved. But choices still have to be made by the therapist to bring the sessions forward. It would be hoped that these are informed choices. In any one session, many things could be transpiring at once in a transference situation. The case of Harvey comes to mind. He was a Vietnam veteran who experienced therapy as an "unmanly" situation. His vivid recollections of the war brought the battlefield and whole armies into the treatment room. His narratives were regularly accompanied by a tightening of his entire musculature so that he had the appearance of a speaking statue. When he allowed himself to come into the therapist's proximity she could feel heat streaming from him. When this was brought to his attention he wanted to know if everybody didn't feel hot when angry. He wanted the therapist out of the way while he thought-murdered a few more enemies. Simultaneously, his eyes glistened as though he were about to cry.

Transferentially, he was in a complex state. He was reliving his experiences in the therapist's presence in such a way as to convey: Help me deal with this. On the other hand, his muscle armor and verbalizations clearly sent a command to stay away. He stated that whatever interventions were offered, they would not make any difference to him. Yet he was close to tears. The therapist finally pointed out how overwrought he was and told him that she would help him sort out how the war affected his present life. She offered herself as someone who could understand his pain. Had the focus been exclusively on one of his many body symptoms, his rigidity, the heat, glistening eyes, and repudiation of help, he would have stayed alone with his horrors.

Instead, he wanted to know how the therapist could tell that along with his anger, he was also uncomfortable. He began to see her as someone who could perhaps walk the long path of recollection with him. Somewhere under all that harshness was a person who could remember emotional contact and closeness after all, and was willing to "transfer" this. Harvey, incidentally, had found his way into movement therapy because he felt that psychiatrists had overmedicated him in an effort to calm him. It was easy to see why some might think he needed tranquilizers. He could hardly sit still and needed to pace and shout frequently. What eventually freed him from his difficulties was the combination of freedom of movement in the sessions and the strong transference he built.

In all therapies, the manner in which transference is dealt with spells either success or failure. Transference is a way of making contact and understanding feelings.

The type of transference anyone is capable of depends on the level of object-relationships while object-relationships in turn are tied to the relative state of the body image. As Schilder (1950) explains, we need the conscious and complete knowledge of our bodies in order to respond fully to others. He states: "A body is necessarily a body among others . . . there is no sense in the word 'ego' when there is no 'thou' "(p. 281). When there is a rigid body and body image, transferences and all mutuality in human relationships suffer.

Schilder gives the *raison dêtre* for dance-movement therapy when he speaks about how the rigid schema of the body loosens during dancing and gymnastics. When we spin rapidly, our perception of the word changes along with the perception of our Selves. While spinning, the world rather than ourselves seems to be in motion. Images blur and we lose our sense of directionality and body boundaries, unless we have learned to "spot." Dancers snap their eyes around to a fixed place while pirouetting in order to forestall the loss of boundaries. But spotting isn't the only dance technique one can either use or discard in order to achieve sensory phenomena. There are many others that can liberate us from our fixed body states. *Grand jétes* or high jumps through space allow us to capture a sensation of soaring through the air; the staccato pounding of a Flamenco can put us in touch with the hauteur of an arrogant aristocrat or the bound sensuality of his lady; a Hula correctly performed can reactivate frozen pelvic rotations and so on. The possibilities are limitless. For people who are not able cognitively to take in complicated dance combinations, an approximation might suffice to stimulate exploration of individual movement styles. This situation is somewhat different for psychotics. Whatever distorted or abbreviated body image exists in them can be totally rigid or it may be so fluid as to incorporate any thing or person. This, of course, is indicative of oral developmental levels. As a matter of course, people whose body image is so uncertain also find it difficult to credit others with firmer identities. Nevertheless, transferences occur.

***

PSYCHOTIC TRANSFERENCE

Psychoanalysts have long broken with Freud's assumption that psychotics are incapable of transference due to their regression to an autoerotic, narcissistic level of development.

The notable success dance-movement therapists often have with psychotic individuals is due largely to their techniques of body-image building and mirroring that allows the fragmented individual to "pull himself together," or, as the British analyst Rosenfeld (1952) states:

> If we avoid attempts to produce positive transference by direct reassurances or expressions of love and simply interpret the positive and negative transferences, the psychotic manifestations attach themselves to the transference in the same way that a transference neurosis develops in a neurotic, there develops what may be called a "transference psychosis"(p. 25).

For the dance-movement therapist, this means that mirroring à la Marianne Chace will reassure the patients that the therapist empathizes with them and will accept them as they are for the time being, without forcing the therapist's own value judgments upon them.

Searles (1963) who worked at Chestnut Lodge, where Marianne Chace also made her discoveries, observes: "The psychotic is so incompletely differentiated in his ego-functioning that he tends to feel not that the therapist reminds him of, or is like, his mother or father (or whomever, from his early life), but rather his functioning is couched in the unscrutinized assumption that the therapist is the mother or father"(p. 252). He also prefers to call these erratic and tenuous interpersonal relationships "Transference Psychosis." For the present purpose, this would be an apt term.

The implications of transference psychosis for any kind of therapist are staggering indeed. Taking on a psychotic individual equals taking on and raising an often physically adult infant. Matters are further complicated as Jacobson (1964) informs us, by the fact that "psychotic patients may develop delusional projective images which they may never attach to definite external persons," and also, that these same patients "may develop delusional self-images which hardly resemble any past or present realistic external objects"(p. 47).

What this means, of course, is that due to his or her distorted or incomplete body image and faulty perception, the psychotic desperately tries to bring some structure and meaning to a destroyed and unfulfilled psychic world.

This structure and meaning is highly egocentric and frequently defies understanding and penetration by the outside world. But their own universe is precious to psychotics. It seems to represent the only proof that they still exist, even if only to themselves. Therefore, they protect themselves with determination.

When even an innocuous "hello" is perceived as a hostile act, swallowed by a boundaryless universe, or dashes to pieces against a disintegrating ego, any therapeutic attempt must at first take the form of creative aggression by the therapist alone.

Margaret Mahler (1968) has chosen the term "Normal Autism" to describe the earliest weeks of life in which the neonate seems to be in "a state of primitive hallucinatory disorientation in which need satisfaction belongs to his own omnipotent, autistic orbit"(p. 7).

This formulation provides a frame of reference. The therapist could offer herself as need-satisfying object to the client who so obviously suffers from an apparent lack of effective tender, loving care.

Isn't the whole state of regression an act expressive of the need to relive and master the time of life in which the trouble first arose, just another side of the prism in the everpresent repetition compulsion?

Freud (1914) thought that we all need to repeat events that overwhelmed us in the past in an effort to master them. This is so in an even more undisguised form for psychotics.

But how does one discern the needs of a nonverbal or totally disoriented person? Does the client live in that rigid state, with those bizarre gestures because of the wish to return to the womb, or the need, at all costs, to control the overwhelming anxiety caused by deneutralized drives, or are both suppositions correct?

Perhaps the client is slightly more advanced, having reached the state of symbiosis which, in Mahler's (1968) terms, means that the "I" and "Not-I" are experienced to be one and the same, that a common boundary exists for both, actually separate, organisms of the mother-child dyad. This kind of behavior would offer the appealing picture of an infant in need.

But why should the clients allow entry into their world on any but their own all-consuming terms? After all, we are never again in life privileged to imagine ourselves so powerful as when we were merged with mother.

The libidinal availability of the mother is another factor that Mahler (1968) stresses, as well as the fact that autonomous ego development and socially adaptive behavior will not emerge unless unpatterned, diffuse and aggressive behavior is counteracted by object love. She states clearly as well that the lack of such object love will often force the deprived infant to turn his aggression against his own body. All this must be remembered by the therapist while the client is busily flicking his wrists, twitching his fingers or merely staring into space. Could this mean "Go away from me," or is it an abreaction of unbearable physical tensions caused by deneutralized aggression flooding the organism?

One way of finding out would be to take the patient's hands into one's own and tell him or her that they are very nice hands. But this may give rise to more anxiety. Suppose the client is not too sure that they are his or her hands, or of flicking them? This person may have withdrawn libidinal cathexis from this area so completely that anesthesia has occurred.

In that event, the therapist's ministrations would only serve to allay her own anxiety and confirm the patient's point of view that there is neither safety nor organization in the world. This kind of approach would have to be postponed until there is some ability on the part of the client to rebuild his or her own body image and its inner representations.

Edith Jacobson (1969) takes another step when she writes that "The infant at first can probably hardly discriminate between his own pleasure sensations and the objects from which they are derived . . . in all probability the child's and his mother's drive-discharge patterns in general become tuned in to each other during the infant's first months of life''(p. 35).

This is very much along the line of thought of Mahler who also recognized that the child will assimilate certain actions and ministrative schemes of the mother during the symbiotic phase but that those assimilations can take place without mental content. Taking in this statement the therapist is now confronted by a client who (1) has broken with reality; (2) needs an all-satisfying source of psychologic and possible material gratification; (3) perhaps does not perceive the self as the person he or she physically and actually is, and (4) has lost objects and their inner representations which never existed except as hallucinations.

Should the therapist now try to interpret what the client might "really" imagine he or she is and respond with action and verbaliztion to this projective image? No. Defining of boundaries and the intrusive thrust of reality will have to be left to a time when the client has already allowed him or her self to be touched by the therapeutic experience.

Would it be feasible intuitively to reproduce the discharge rhythms of the client's early infancy to enable acceptance of the therapist as a substitute parent? Hardly, since in all likelihood, arhythmicity existed between the mothering figure and the client in early infancy. At first it is impossible to pick up correctly and understand schizophrenic "babylike" clients' signals. Observation will gradually facilitate some understanding and open the door for intervention.

Jacobson (1969) further postulates that during the progress of a psychosis as well as during certain psychosomatic diseases, there might be a "decrease in the cathexes of the periphery, of perceptive and motor functions, resulting in the rise of the cathexes of the body organs, with concomitant regressive drive defusion to the point of prevalence of destructive drive energy which again must be discharged through the physiological channels in the body''(p. 17).

Observing the grimacing of some schizophrenic clients, the inward-turned gaze and lanquid smile so reminiscent of the neonate, the therapist might try picking up ''clues'' and ask simple questions. For instance, a twenty year-old woman, Eve, obviously had to go to the bathroom. She grimaced and squirmed exactly like a baby about to defecate into its diapers. The therapist's simple question: ''Do you want to go to the bathroom?'' was received as an affirmation of her magical powers and of Eve's transparency. She became panic-stricken because she was sure the therapist could actually see through her physically. The therapist's support was simply not experienced as such. Leaving her in discomfort until she might have found the necessary words herself could have been more beneficial. Having to inform the therapist that she had to leave the room would have been an object-related act.

To phrase it differently, even a simple ''hello'' accompanied by a smile meaning ''I am here with you,'' could appear to clients as a perpetuation of what they already know, namely, that nobody understands them.

An example comes to mind in which a severely regressed boy, Bob, darted anxiously into a corner every time I said ''hello'' upon entering his classroom in a special school. He was willing to shake hands, however, in direct contradiction, I then thought, of the immense concrete importance usually given by schizophrenics to words. The rest of the people in the class did say ''hello,'' and having incorporated me with this acknowledgement into their generally boundless world, were content to ignore me after that, while Bob had to shake hands in order to accomplish the same obliteration. He would cautiously emerge from his corner, shake hands, and then completely ignore all of us.

After about 6 months of intensive work, when all the others in the group where already eagerly looking forward to their movement therapy sessions, Bob still confined his actions to the handshake and darting into the corner. Winter was upon us. I was late one morning and rushed into the session, still feeling cold. Bob shook hands with me, as usual. But instead of leaving in a headlong lunge, he stayed glued to the spot, and kept pumping my hand. Finally, he said: "Your hands are cold. I am cold." I was able to use the concept of the conflict-free ego sphere here, although my interpersonal formulations so far had not been helpful. At least Bob's thermal apparatus was still intact. I therefore embarked on a course of examing temperature differences with Bob. We felt walls and found them to be hard and cold. So were furniture and floors. Radiators were hard and warm. Did that mean they were alive? Following Bob's initiative, we began to ask people's permission to touch them. Bob figured out that people are hard and soft, cold and warm, and so was his therapist! Could that mean that he, Bob, had all these properties? Animate and inanimate became concepts to Bob which he tested again and again.

At this time, he told me that in the beginning when I so cheerfully greeted him and his group by saying "hello," he only heard "hell." He felt sure then that I would send him and his peers to hell. He saw my cheerfulness as evidence that I would do so since obviously so much cheer must be a sign that I had a lot of power. Bob's verbal communications alerted me to the fact that in the past his hearing had been affected by his psychological problems. Certainly he had no difficulties in hearing completely what was said after he was able to tell me so much. His teacher also commented on his increased alertness and ability to attend. It can be seen how useful the concept of the conflict-free ego-sphere was in this application, even though in Bob's case it had been so constricted that only single apparati were available for interaction. Nonetheless, even with so little available to him, Bob formed at first a negative, than a positive transference to me, in a fusing mode. At first, he assumed that he must be cold because I was. I have often wondered if he also felt I would go to hell with him! Bob was not the only one whose fluctuating transference state gave me pause.

The difficulty with these clients in dance-movement therapy is that one day they wish to cling and be rocked, they ask for unending body contact and their therapist's eternal presence, while on the next day they stare with vacant eyes at the "mother-therapist" of yesterday. This withdrawal is a protective device, designed to spare the client acknowledgement of the repeated separations from the therapist.

Another illustration of such a case is Donna, who was upset when the therapist had to be absent from her sessions. The intern who substituted correctly picked up Donna's anxiety, which manifested itself in tremors in arms and legs and quick hopping from one foot to the next. Donna kept asking where the bird was and what had happened to the tail. The intern led the group into a dance of birds flying. Most of the group members enjoyed it but Donna's anxiety increased. She kept searching the room for the "bird" and did not quiet down until I resumed the sessions. It was then possible to establish that to Donna "Siegel" had become "seagull" who had disappeared and left the poor little tail, Donna, all alone. As soon as this was correctly understood, Donna was able to quiet down and even to use "Seagull's" absence and return as a learning experience that gave her confidence enough to let her mother and teacher leave without protest, once she had recognized these women as significant also. This did not take place until after the episode described.

This illustration of the severe body image distortion in a fourteen year-old girl is quite typical for this level of development. It approximates the "eight month's anxiety" Spitz describes in infants, who at that age are loath to be with strangers and wish to stay close to mother. The normal infant, of course, does not imagine itself to be the tail of a bird, or, indeed, that its mother is a bird. Donna had so far left reality that an attachment to a real person had become too dangerous, and a seagull seemed safer.

A useful exercise with this kind of person is to balance balloon sticks between the flattened upright hands of client and therapist and to have the client lead the therapist, and vice versa, by gentle directional pressure. Music can be appropriately used since it gives an additional structure to the "leading each other." This reinforces reality perception because the sense of touch is isolated from actual body contact. Client and therapist are close in this exercise, but not so close that the threat of merger and total loss of self re-engulfs the patient.

Donna's level of development and transference response are already beyond two other types frequently encountered.

Autistic Transference Manifestations

The first is the autistic one, the total unawareness of another-than-self. Developmentally this is linked with the first weeks of life. Neonates are also totally unaware of their environment until the ministering, stroking and need-gratification by the mother eventually makes them aware of another-than-self that finally turns out to be "Mother." The body image slowly forms as Mother caresses her child and gives it adequate care. As infants experience themselves, they also learn about the hand that strokes them and the breast that feeds them. The neonate in the nursing position feels mother's warmth, her breathing rhythm, and her skin surface. As the infant's body image becomes more complete, so does the infant's perception of the "significant object"—Mother.

Confronted by the Autist of whatever age it is often necessary to abandon the usual approach technique of dance-movement therapy, which is mirroring. Because mirroring relies so heavily on the visual reception of the client, the therapist is frequently unperceived. Mirroring as an approach technique with autists depends on their visual acuity, not only on their willingness or unwillingness to make contact. Bob's functional impairment of the auditory sphere has been described. The same encroachment upon vision might have prevented Sherry, Danny, Joe, Pete, and many others from responding. They simply could not look at their therapist mirroring them.

Ruttenberg (1971) conceptualizes that autists at first

transverse a pre-oral, sensorimotor stage in which un-modulated, erratic motility and unstable sensory reception predominate. Piaget (1972) recognizes such an early sensorimotor phase in life and believes it to be the most creative in a person's life. He also believes it to continue until the emergence of speech. For the autist no such Piagetian creativity can take place. They are incredibly concrete in what they perceive, if they perceive at all. For instance, they may know what a fork is but believe only the one fork they use always to be a fork. No other utensils of the same shape are recognized as what they are. Piagetian meaning-giving and reflective abstraction does not take place.

Spitz' (1965) concept of a phase in which reflexive learning is the order of the day is applicable here. During the well-documented first 3 months of life all perceiving and learning has the nature of a conditioned reflex and only secondarily takes on psychologic meaning when pleasure and unpleasure are connected with stimulus responses. Due to the immaturity of the sensorium, we must first learn to use our ego apparati in a life-sustaining manner. Although we hear, see, smell, feel, we cannot organize the received stimuli into meaningful constructs until the duality of physical maturation and psychological development enables us to do so.

Autistic clients can be likened to neonates in the reflexive phase, even when they are as large as the therapist, or larger. They are stuck in the area of contact perception in which shapes and people and things merge into fused and shifting forms that are not reliably constant. We all rely on contact perception at birth, until our maturing sensorium allows us to judge distance perception to be more constant. It is easy to lose the image of mother's face in nondifferentiation and to rely on smell or touch at first. But later, eyes can follow mother even from the crib, so that distance perception is reinforced by its longer reach.

The autists discussed here were not measurably organically impaired. But they did not, and could not, look at their therapist mirroring them, nor did they allow themselves to be touched.

This observation is in opposition to Rutter's (1979) view that autists do allow close physical proximity. To Rutter and his colleagues the superficial "learned" hugs and acquienscence to bodily manipulating produced by behavior modification techniques constitute body contact. In the psychoanalytic frame of reference, however, the quality of such touching is of foremost importance.

For instance, when a child or adult uses the therapist's hands to acquire a needed toy for the first time, is a sign that the client is not yet able to trust all of the therapist. When that same person begins to snuggle up to the therapist without looking, a big step has been taken toward establishing a more complete interpersonal relationship. Many of the movement sessions with these clients take place on the floor. Upright posture and meaningful locomotion belong to another developmental level, even though most can and do walk with varying speed, and appear to have acquired some rudimentary sense of space.The word "rudimentary" is used advisedly here because it is not an uncommon occurrence, nor is stepping on a classmate who is sitting quietly, but happens to be in the way.

Bobby's behavior illustrates this. His conscientious teacher spent many hours dangling a small ball in front of him which he was supposed to follow with his eyes. Sometimes he did and sometimes he didn't. The teacher was quite convinced that Bobby was manipulating her with his erratic attendance. But the blank look on Bobby's face spoke of a self-immersion so deep that it was doubtful he was even aware of her. He was willing enough to come to his movement sessions—though "willing" is not quite the right word—he was simply uninterested. I sang to him, imitating his long, low ululations. Sometimes, when he appeared to look at me fleetingly I mirrored him. He, however, spent his time gazing impassively into nowhere. Sometimes he ululated. At other times he would whirl a small toy.

I had only one clue that he was really aware of what was going on: he became very upset if I did not play music. Others among his classmates were fascinated by the record player itself.

Not so Bobby. He wanted to hear music and began to scream if this was withheld. His teachers used music as a reward for compliance or performance of a task. I felt reluctant to use the same technique but I did observe that Bobby would look at me directly when he wanted music. I used this fleeting contact over and over again to say "Which music do you want, Bobby?" Eventually, I was rewarded. Bobby grabbed my hand and put it on the record of his choice. We were both pleased with this interaction. Bobby gave one of his secret smiles that vanished the second he thought someone saw it. Eventually, he began to bring his own records from the classroom with him and the two of us sat and listened. It was during one of these quiet interludes that Bobby, who was sitting at some distance from me on the floor, suddenly scooted across the floor on his behind and landed himself in my lap with aplomb. It took much longer before he could stand in front of me and give me a hug. Individuals who immediately respond to touch and body contact are probably only secondarily autistic, having regressed from the symbiotic phase when the demands fo maturation and development became too threatening for their fragile egos.

After working with many Bobbys and observing the similarities in their nonresponses and wardings-off, I devised some techniques in order to help us build our tenous base of a transference more readily.

Lying down on the floor alongside the client, both therapist and client on their sides and facing each other will produce a simple finger game. Fingers might simply touch, or hands might move together. Actually, this is a form of mirroring as well, because the random hand-movements of the client are picked up and either directed or shaped by both. Not surprisingly, there is almost always eye contact in this position. It feels indeed like gazing into the profound stare of a neonate.

Another structured game is best used after the finger-play, when transference manifestations of a primitive nature have already surfaced.

Those autistic or presymbiotic individuals, in whom the aggressive drive predominates, often allow themselves to become aware of pleasure as opposed to constant displeasure when it is made safe for them to lie down flat on their backs, placing their feet on the therapist's shoulders and pushing and bending their knees. Initially the clients' knees may fall open and muscle tremor occur while the face assumes a distant, vacant look. Drooling and thumb-sucking may be resorted to in order to block out the presence of this intruding other-than-self. However, this exercise has multiple purposes. It provides a chance to organize erratic motility while discharging aggression in a safe way in the push against the therapist's shoulders. When the tremors in the legs are too strong, or the knees merely fall open in avoidance of the push, leaning down a little more heavily so that the therapist's weight can be felt and holding the knees in place help the client gather up enough intent for a good push. Needless to say, the therapist can fly clear across the room when the person in question is too strong.

Ideally, a rhythmic pushing is produced that has the therapist bobbing up and down with the client's feet firmly on her shoulders. Most of the time, though, memory traces of being diapered and taken care of appear to be reactivated and the first signs of true transference manifestations begin to occur. After this intervention people like Bobby can be found prone on the floor, legs up, ready for the exercises. Usually, the client also begins to stare at the therapist's face and between solid pushes against her shoulders ventures a smile or reaches out toward her face; in short, what was not feasible in the libidinal position of being rocked and caressed becomes attainable when a restructured outlet for aggression is provided.

Secondarily autistic persons will benefit by sitting on the floor between the therapist's legs in front of a mirror. Gentle background music can provide an added stimulus to raising and lowering arms together. The therapist provides the intial "motor" and doing it for the client. Bending and stretching of legs in the same position often affords the hyperactive runner as well as the withdrawn dreamer an opportunity to lean against the therapist's physical and emotional availability. This facilitates the giant step toward symbiosis.

Another factor that aids in establishing transference is a simple technique called "Breathing Together." I had noticed for a long while that almost none of the regressed people I worked with were able to draw a deep breath when it was appropriate to do so. Even after relatively strenuous exercise they would not inhale deeply. Under ordinary circumstances, their breathing patterns always seemed shallow and arhythmic. As research eventually proved quite conclusively, the psychotic children I worked with did not regulate their breathing apparatus in the same fashion as others. They use only 1/3 of their Forced Vital Capacity (Siegel & Blau, 1978) so that their bodies are forever deprived of the needed amounts of oxygen.

Although breathing is an autonomous reflex, Blau and I have hypothesized that it is also connected with psychophysiologic systems. For instance, the neonate adapts its breathing rhythms to that of the mother. A synchronicity evolves that paves the way for other tasks of living within the human community. When mother and child do not evolve this synchronicity, maladaptation forms. Kestenberg (1967) has shown that scrutiny of body rhythms can help to forecast whether a mother-child dyad will pass through all phases with favorable results or not. In "Breathing Together," Blau and I conceptualized the breathing apparatus as being connected with the formation of the first body ego and body image. Once the need for survival has forced the first independent breath upon the neonate, breathing patterns must be adapted to those of the mother. While being held, the baby quite literally feels if the mother is anxiously sucking in her breath, or expelling it forcefully in anger, or if she is breathing peacefully and contentedly. Her innate patterns will always prevail in whatever emotional state and give the baby clues on how to adapt. In oversimplified terms, this is part of the process of bonding between mother and child which makes them a psychologic unit. At the same time, the baby learns about is own body while it becomes larger with a deep breath and pushes against mother, or draws away when inhaling.

It has already been noted that characteristics of autistic

clients are reminisent of these early states. Therefore, "Breathing Together" with them seemed a phase-specific kind of activity tending to create the climate necessary for transference. It is a simple technique. I place my hand on the chest of the client and he or she reciprocates. Even if the client is nonverbal, I reassure him or her that the air is good for both of us. Then I try to pick up the other's breathing rhythm. Often this is so shallow and erratic that I have a hard time not to gasp. When I feel the client relaxing into our togetherness, I say: "Try it my way now." At first, not much might happen. After many sessions, a steady rhythmic rocking emerges that expresses our breathing together comfortably and easily. This is another step toward the formation of a true transference relationship.

But there are some who are even more difficult to reach. In their defensive withdrawal from any human contact they have erected such a formidable fortification that they are quite often regarded as untreatable. However, it is their defense that is autistic, not their total selves. In working with classically autistic people, the absence of symbolization in the beginning phases of treatment is striking. Actually, symbolization does not occur until about three months of age. (Deutsch, 1959; Spitz 1965). But in the individuals described below, symbolization is strongly developed. Indeed, understanding their symbolizations is the key that unlocks the heavily guarded doors of their minds for transference.

This type of client is rarely seen in private practice. The depth of their regression precludes even minimal participation in family life or work. To take on such clients means that the therapist could find herself reconstructed as magic eye, a chair, or a turnip. Anything is possible once the therapist is caught up by the whirlpool of these clients' unneutralized agression. Unneutralized aggression is perhaps not the right term although it is used often enough when talking about these clients. Their aggression has turned both against the self and others; they appear to distrust themselves and others to an incredible degree.

Neutralization is a hypothetical psychic process whereby unbound, destructive drive energy becomes modified and tamed through the medium of interpersonal relationships. The process of neutralization, or making both aggressive and libidinal drive energy useful, is significantly linked with normal development. As the baby realizes that there is no need to scream furiously, because food and nurturing are provided by mother, it can give up the overwhelming tensions that flood it and begin to turn its attention toward the bringer of good feelings and the self. When there is a failure in this process from either side of the dyad, faulty ego and superego formation occurs.

The clients who have not been able to cope with their aggression and have not been able to gentle it through taking in what care was provided for them will sometimes end with the kind of thick wall between themselves and the universe that is said to be autistic. Those among them who develop a new set of bizarre behavior patterns once treatment starts are obviously more "with it" and somewhat more reachable than those who are stoically bent upon perpetuating their nothingness.

However, even those people to whom "nothingness" is the most precious defense of all, often in varying degrees bestow upon their therapist the pent-up fury of their incompletely neutralized energies so that the therapist by figuratively keeping her head above the storm, i.e. keeping calm and neutral toward the onslaught of the patient's rage, may achieve a starting point for contact and transference.

Clients who have one steady formula for expressing everything, from perception of proprioceptive stimuli to anger at their attendants to love for themselves are the most difficult. Transference manifestatins of any kind seem to be absent, as hour after hour the client babbles the same set of words or performs the same combination of gross and fine motor acts.

The meaning of such sequences is exceedingly difficult to penetrate since they are used multiply. They apparently have lost their usual symbolic meaning, much as objects have lost their boundaries in the patient's psyche. But these appearances are deceptive. The symbolisms have been so condensed and adjusted by clients' unconscious needs that they serve both to express meaning and to fend off any understanding of their meanings. If jumping up and down and pointing to the ceiling while shouting "at statue, a statue" today means "I have an erection", tomorrow it might mean "Please go away." Verbal interpretation is usually warded off completely or incorporated in such a fashion that it reinforces the motor stimulus and becomes part of the defensive reenactment of the stereotyped behavior. Mirroring is ignored.

In the example cited above a chronically schizophrenic boy of fourteen had used the jumping and pointing while shouting "A statue, a statue" as his sole form of expression for 4 years. Even when heavily sedated he would periodically rouse himself to perform his special act. Not much was known of his previous history. According to the record, he had always been "odd." His parents claimed to have already known that he was ill when they were told that he was schizophrenic at age six. He was then placed in a special class in public school. He learned to read but was admitted to a school for special children when he was ten and the above described pattern began to predominate. Shortly thereafter, he was hospitalized.

By observing in minutest details how he used his particular formula, it became possible to understand his daily performance, but both attempts at interpretation and at direct confrontation with the contents of his action made no impression. On rare occasions they influenced him to reel off his stereotyped chant at terrific speed. Apparently at such times, even in this deeply withdrawn boy, inexact interpretation forced his one functioning pseudo-defense to deepen.

After many months, this boy's attendant began to complain that Dave would no longer sit still and do his puzzles and word games as he used to but would jump, point, and shout at regular intervals all day instead of just occasionally. He would become especially excited when his therapist was slated to appear. I felt agitated myself when I saw how frantically Dave performed his stereotyped recitation. Because my appearance seemed to exacerbate it, I decided to interpret it as a transference reaction. When Dave next did his frenzied jump-point-shout formula, I said "You think I give you permission to jump and tell about the statue." He immediately came to a full stop and allowed himself to look at me directly.

Little by little, fragments of what he was trying to say emerged. Dave drew a huge picture on the wall that reached from floor to ceiling. He identified this picture as "the dead Dave" and jumped up high to touch the head of the drawing. I offered him a chair to stand on, but that was too easy for Dave. He told me that his dead self was also much larger than the self that was standing there and that he had to catch it in order to make it smaller and managable again. He had to turn it into a statue which was not alive and therefore not dangerous. The jumping and pointing was related to this body image distortion in which he felt himself so much larger than life that he had to declare himself dead. The thought "I am aware of the therapist outside of myself" appeared to activate tensions which were released physically for the therapist as a primitive seduction, an approach device, and a renewed attempt to construct boundaries. This was deduced from the fact that Dave did stop in front of the therapist instead of running her down during his performance, something he often did to attendants and aides.

The spacing and timing of his sterotype became his specific transference manifestation. He eventually verbalized that he believed everybody but the therapist and himself to be either dead or from "up there," the top of his split-off dead self and the world which he perceived as above and on top of himself. Later, short, interpretive questions such as "What are you standing on?" or "Where are your feet right now?" served to reinforce a rudimentary form of reality testing when Dave was able to answer them directly. These questions also brought about a diminution of excitement as Dave began to perceive himself more realistically.

SYMBIOTIC "CLINGING" TRANSFERENCE

Once clients have allowed themselves the union of symbiosis, an entirely different motor behavior takes shape. They readily and easily pick up any form of dance or rhythm presented, but seem incapable of improvising any but the most primitive patterns on their own. When the therapist is not visually available, the clients fall back on their unstructured earlier mode of locomotion and seem to have forgotten what was gained during therapy. The therapist's libidinal as well as physical availability more than once a week is essential here to produce enough of an interpersonal relationship to establish a true transference psychosis. During this phase much work can be done on body image. Clients need to feel the therapist's face and perhaps the entire periphery of her body and must learn the limits of how much touching is comfortable and acceptable, both to themselves and to the therapist. In other words, the mutual tactile explorations must be kept within limits to allow for neutralization of drives.

When it is totally inappropriate to touch each other, tracing each other's outline on large rolls of brown paper is a good device. Upon completion of this task, the client is asked to use a crayon or chalk to fill in the details of facial features and clothing. Not surprisingly, pictures often turn out to have the same haircut and to wear the same skirt, regardless of sex difference. Symbiosis truly means experiencing two people as one. That is why it is so important to provide boundaries and to set limits. Symbiotic people often like to stay in their sessions forever. Time is not experienced as a concept that can be useful. As one of my clients said: "I think there must be two kinds of time. One that staff people use and one that patient people use. Staff people chop up time and make mincemeat out of it. Patient people make taffy out of it so it becomes sweet and lasts forever." At the time he delivered his thoughtul message to me he was trying to persuade me to let him "be boss of when the sessions end."

His statement was rather more sophisticated than those of others who simply refuse to leave when the time has come or find that they have remembered a dream, or want to demonstrate a dance that just occurred to them. Another group needs to be held and rocked, no matter how "grown-up" they are. I have held and rocked grandmothers whose lives had deprived them of all they loved until they themselves became helpless infants in hospitals, I have rocked veterans of two wars whose martial deeds had haunted them into denial of reality, and I have rocked little children who were finally ready to accept an other-than-self into their universe. They had this in common: the need to relive for an instant the concrete reality of another human being they could incorporate without danger and with whom they could identify. They also, very simply, needed to consolidate their own body images by learning from me what a body is like.

BORDERLINE VACILLATIONS

The transference situation becomes considerably more complex when the separation-individuation phase of development has been reached. Normally, the child has learned to say "no" at this time and experiments extensively with this new power. The toddler plays for a while, then returns for emotional refueling. The baby-client experiments similarly with the treatment situation. Resistances become more complex. They may be a constant vacillation between meaningful expressive movements, teasing, a desire to change places with the therapist, and anger at being mirrored. Mirroring at this phase is often experienced as being made fun of. The client needs a period of dancing by her or himself for the empathetic and admiring therapist-audience. At the same time there may be whole sessions in which it is necessary for therapist and client at first to sit companionably with each other and do no more than look at each other fully or to wind up breathing rhythmically together. It is as though the blossoming wholeness growing in the client needs to be filled with the essence of the therapist-mother so that the essential merger will never be forgotten again.

But before this happy event can take place, many contradictory transference phases have to be lived through.

"Vacillation" is the key word for the recognition of the Borderline Personality. Quite literally, the adored person of today becomes tomorrow's object of ridicule and hate. This then also manifests itself in the transference and is difficult to cope with. Psychoanalytic theoreticians hypothesize that the mechanism of splitting enables people afflicted by a Borderline Personality Organization to keep opposite perceptions of one and the same person separate.

Kohut (1971, 1977) and Kernberg (1975, 1976) have identified two subgroups whose symptoms are similar. They have suffered a critical wound to their narcissism so that instead of healthy self-esteem, grandiosity and an inability to form appropriate interpersonal relationships appears. The inner representations of an other-than-self are hazy and commingled with unrealistic perceptions of the self. Kohut uses the word "selfobject" to delineate a form of inner object representation that isn't quite as diffuse or distorted as those in psychotics but bears some of the same hallmarks.

In the group Kernberg describes, rage at having been consistently misunderstood and disappointed predominates. Such individuals seek isolation and flight in order to keep themselves intact. (Stolorow & Lachman, 1980). A homeostasis is maintained which balances opposing views of the same person. The borderline persons misperceptions of their surrounding world is not as profound as that of psychotics. The boundaries between themselves and the important people in their lives are not as destroyed. They are simply more rigorously defended. Anxiety is always high in case an other-than-self will intrude.

Morton was a person who gloried in his "self-sufficiency." After announcing with certainty that he needed a movement therapist, he flung himself on the couch in the classic position and from there began to harangue the therapist upon the lack of conceptualization in dance-movement therapy and her own shortcomings, i.e. he undid his own intent by making her into an analyst. It soon became clear that he was repeating a long-standing behavior pattern. Just as we were about to investigate this supposition, he switched his stance. He wanted the therapist to dance for him and promised he would follow along. A period of flattery and attempts at seduction ensued. This showed clearly that Morton was interested in only one thing: to manipulate the therapist according to his own needs.

During this largely verbal production he frequently changed color. He grew pale with rage when his wishes weren't followed and blushed with shame when he did not find his offers of dates, theatre tickets, and flowers accepted. During this time, his breathing pattern was highly constricted and erratic and there was no mobility in his upper torso. When he turned to the therapist, he did so with his entire body, never just from the waist. There was also a stiffness in the way he carried his head. Head and shoulders moved in a unit. Yet this same man was quite capable of performing complex Tai Chi sequences which he learned in order to show the therapist how wrong her approach was in his opinion.

The contradictions in Morton's behavior, both physical and psychologic, were self-evident. They bore similarity to the way another client, Madge, behaved. Yet the reasons for Madge's splitting were entirely different. She appeared as unable as Morton to form a stable and close transference relationship. But her life history disclosed something akin to a developmental arrest in the area of her self-esteem. Kohut sees such people as having been treated without empathy by their surroundings. They are not unloved, merely totally misunderstood. In Madge's case, her mother was so preoccupied with her own needs that she didn't notice when Madge tried to behave in a specially pleasing way or dressed herself in clothes she thought mother would approve of. Her mother was an actress who related to the child as though she were a puppy. She consistently misread Madge's attempts at pleasing as showing off. Despite such repeated disappointments, Madge, like all children, needed to love her mother. In an effort not to feel the pain of prolonged rebuttal, she identified with Mother or anyone else who came along who held out the promise of security and love. In this way she could share in other people's glory and needed none of her own. Once she entered treatment the therapist found it hard to believe at first that this clinging vine was also a high-powered fashion model who often outdid her peers in assignments. However, the day when the therapist fell from her pedestal in Madge's eyes came soon enough. She thought that the therapist failed to appreciate sufficiently her "wonderful" photographer friend. This was enough to send her into sulky silence and inactivity when before she could not do enough to assure the therapist that she always "made her feel better with her gentleness."

Both Morton and Madge were like the young child who thinks his Mommy is bad when she refuses to give out cookies indiscriminately. And of course the same Mommy is also the best in the world when her actions coincide with her child's wishes. It takes a lot of maturation and development before the child can acknowledge that his mother and others are both good and bad.

In the transferences, these contradictions are reproduced. In motility they are expressed as variously as in the feeling states of the clients. Some days these people are able to do everything superbly, the next day they assume the plaintive helplessness of someone who can barely locomote. It all has an "as if" quality (Deutsch, 1942) which makes all therapeutic gains questionable.

THE STUBBORN TRANSFERENCES IN OBSESSION COMPULSION

The deep split betwen psyche and soma observed in this type of neurosis responds readily to a somewhat more sophisticated form of dance-movement therapy than simply mirroring and body-image building. However, since obsessional clients are a good deal further along the developmental scale and command a more complex aresenal of resistances, interpersonal relationships, and perceptions, it is even more important to zero in on transferences and to "do" something about them. Obsessional clients are not nearly so indifferent as the autistic, nor so dependent as the symbiotic. In contrast to the Borderline, they obstinately hang on to their opinions about the therapist and everything else, despite evidence that they might be in error. Indeed, they may be proud of their "independence" and walk out of a session never to return if negative transferences are not dealt with on time. Since all their behavior is marked by a deep ambivalence, with emotional coldness and hostility surfacing frequently, they are often mistaken for a borderline personality organization or vice versa. Even highly skilled diagnosticians cannot always differentiate these states sufficiently to forecast a definitive prognosis at the beginning of treatment.

In borderline states, there is a tendency to give way to psychotic aspects under stress since defenses are unevolved and interpersonal relationships shallow. Flexibility and adaptability are greatly reduced so that transferences also are brittle and shallow. The obsessive-compulsive person, is however, capable of strong attachments and of making a neurotic transference. Psychosexually, he is fixated on the anal-sadistic level, or as several clients observed wryly, they are "stuck in the shit period." The preoccupation with feces is evident not only in psychological rigidity and often exaggerated fear of death but in tightened sphincter muscles, overly erect posture and an inability simply to "enjoy" anything. Any encroachment on their ritualistic ways is met with an increase in anxiety, attempts at undoing, and isolation.

The opposite of all these characteristics falls into the same nosologic category, such as the slovenly person who thinks it is too bad that other people cannot tolerate the stench from his or her unwashed body. This kind of overt obsessional person may show up in dirty clothes reeking from old perspiration and meet interpretive questions as to why he or she needs to overpower with smell with the answer: "What's the matter? You compulsive or something? Washing is just a foolish convention thought up by the establishment to sell more soap."

It is important to maintain neutrality with such clients. They are completely capable of making their own choices. They merely need a catalyst in the person of the therapist to deflect unresolved conflict.

In normal development there is, during the anal phase, a marked emergence of the aggressive drive, admixed with the libidinal and sadistic impulses; sphincter control is achieved, and passivity gives way to activity. At the same time, ambivalence toward the mother arises in the struggle for individuation. Anal eroticism forms, with all its concomitant pleasures in olfactory sensations, withholding and expelling.

The fixations formed at this time of life are readily recognized in the behavior of these clients. They both love and hate the therapist but always with the awareness that this is an advanced and beneficial form or make-believe. The anally oriented client never makes the mistake of confusing the therapist with the real-life persons in his or her early life.

Displacement of tension from one set of muscles to another is often present in the obsessive-compulsive client. While constipation and rigid sphincters are a regular accompaniment, this can also be displaced to arhythmic breathing patterns, unduly rigid shoulder girdle or lack of pelvic swing. Unlike the psychotic patient who clings and cannot separate from the therapist once a transference occurs, the obsessional will undo the pleasure of loosening up and breathing freely either by denying that results are being obtained or by claiming that they do not matter. As these clients' improvisations become more spontaneous and their use of space less constricted, a simultaneous moving away from the therapist will take place. They say: "Surely you are trying to control me secretly and magically. You only make believe that my spurt of growth is desirable!"

In other words, the improvisations express both the client's wish to be healthy and the morbid suspicion that it is not possible for him to attain emotional health. Fear of being controlled and manipulated is countered by paying fees late or not at all and by not acknowledging the visible signs of success. Sadistic impulses are acted upon in this controlling and withholding way, testing the therapists patience and skill until the disappointments and frustrations of early life have been sufficiently explored and integrated. During this period of working through, the body stance of the client often reveals a "toddler's pose." Torso and hips are used as one unit, with abdomen thrust forward, a hollow spine, and flattened feet planted solidly into the ground. Preferred movement pattern are abandoned for flailing arms and a stamping, heavy gait in order to re-experience the defiance necessary for individuation.

This is a transitory stage. Torso and hips are never fused with the same solidity as in psychosis. Frequently such clients have an active sex life and even experience orgasm physiologically. However, they become easily bored with their partners and tend to blame them for the lack of true orgasmic pleasure, just as the therapist is blamed for lack of "progress." Once the toddler's body stance gives way to the motility of a maturing individual, a blossoming of intelligence, creativity, a true ability to love and enjoy life takes place that can only be described as amazing. All the energy hitherto bound by ritualistic "no-saying" to the world, withholding, and magic thinking begins to serve the client to the extent that he or she can begin to see the therapist as a real person from whom it is possible to separate without hostility or fear of reprisal. From the above discussion it can easily be seen that most of the transference in the treatment of obsessive-compulsive individuals is marked by both physiologic and psychologic negativism, or, at best, ambivalence.

THE CLASSIC TRANSFERENCE

The kind of pathology connected with fixation to the next phase in psychosexual development and maturation is the phallic one. Psychoanalysis offers a good-to-excellent prognosis for these patients referred to as "hysteric." Although there are often acute physical symptoms, the more complex and nearly complete state of object-relationships and largely intact ego of the hysteric can readily make use of verbal interpretations.

Despite this fact, people who fall into this diagnositc category gravitate toward dance-movement therapy also. Perhaps they are the ones whose strong motor drive prevents them from accepting the prone position on the couch in analysis for any length of time. They are not always as easy to work with as their high developmental level suggests. Frequently they have learned to deal with their difficulties by ignoring them. This emotional distancing of necessity also occurs in the treatment situation. If conversion symptoms are present, they are denied or are dealt with as a physical illness.

Conversions are physiologic manifestations without physiologic causes. Typically, the hysterical client refuses to believe the doctor's dictum that there is nothing amiss when cramp, anesthesias, paralysis, or tremors occur. Sometimes there are emotional spells during which consciousness is temporarily altered. Amnesia is also a major concern.

Jolinda's case is an illustration of all the factors mentioned. She came to dance-movement therapy with a multiplicity of bodily symptoms. The most conspicuous one was the way she carried her left arm, bent and close to her body. She treated her arm as though it were a silly nuisance and made brave little jokes about her "crippler." A long series of physical treatments had brought her little relief. She entered analysis but left again to seek this therapist out because her ex-analyst, according to her, was "charming, a good man who didn't understand about arms."

Jolinda worked diligently but always excluded her arm from movement. Finally, during an improvisation in which she saw herself as saving a drowning child, she reached out with both arms. Apparently, she was totally unaware that she was doing so. I quickly grabbed her hand and held her arm in the fully stretched position she herself had adopted. The emotional thunderstorm that followed was of gigantic proportions. Small wonder, I had deprived Jolinda of her cherished, masochistic fantasy that she was a cripple. It took a long time to work through all the ramifications of this incident. Had it not been for Jolinda's strong transference, my intervention surely would have been too intrusive. As it was, she could not help but see me as her rescuer. As such, I had usurped her own role in the fantasy. She felt that it was herself she was saving but also, that it was "undignified" to need rescue at all.

The special kinds of transferences that arise during depression, phobias, and conversion are also subject to interpretation according to developmental level. A psychotic person can also be depressed, have phobias, and suffer from conversions. It is the high level of steady interpersonal relationships that identifies the so-called hysteric.

Quite obviously, working with many people on an indepth level arouses feelings inside of the therapist, too. These are the ubiquituous countertransferences.

COUNTERTRANSFERENCE IN DANCE-MOVEMENT THERAPY

Experience has shown that countertransferences are deeper and need to be monitored more closely in dance-movement therapy than in psychoanalysis. In mirroring their clients physically, dance-movement therapists regularly and in each session make a "trial identification" with them that is bound to leave its residual echo. A psychoanalyst's trial identification involves a volitional act in which she opens herself up totally for a short span of time during any one session in order to capture her analysand's essence. But a dance-movement therapist does not really have a choice in the matter. She must pick up movement clues as they are presented to her. In doing so, she cannot help but identify with her clients as she receives physically through imitation their moods, intent, and defenses along with their motility. Leaving all this on the unspoken level can arouse strange reverberations in the therapist. Pacing along with an agitated client is quite simply agitating, feeling the tentative touch of a frightened child is saddening: theses experiences are manifold and cannot be escaped. This physical, imitative experiencing of another's movements fosters not only "knowing," them but unconscious identifications. If these identifications are not immediately brought to the surface and dealt with they distort and overlay the therapist's own motility. No amount of training can prepare one adequately for the first shock of unwanted and unsolicited contact with the murderous rage of a client as it plows into the hidden oedipal recesses of the unwary therapist. Therapists obviously have to learn how to deal with stimuli received from clients in their own therapy.

As supervisor I have observed again and again that neophyte therapists who are not yet in therapy themselves may be able to read their own countertransferential body signals correctly, but they do not know what to do with them. This is especially true when working with autistic and psychotic clients.

When becoming aware of the annihilating fear or hate in clients, one needs to remind oneself that it is they who fear death and mutilation, not oneself. The same is true when symbiotic clients try to engulf their therapist with their most flowery fancies. But being aware is not enough. After a session in which someone has literally burrowed his head into my lap and sobbed, or has attempted to take me in so completely that I feel drained, I need to give myself a movement experience that puts me back in touch with my own body ego. For me, this is most often a dance class or the execution of a simple exercise on the ballet barre in my studio. As I feel my own muscles relax in a stretch and my spine flexibly erect over my center, the countertransferential distress lessens and I begin to move again in the mode that is organic for me. After this I can empathize with clients much more readily.

I have known therapists who instead of searching for their strengths thought they needed relaxation after a strenuous bout with agitated psychotic clients. They sought out saunas and massages and came back deliciously relaxed but also totally vulnerable in their muscular relaxation to the renewed onslaught by their clients.

When the symbolic threat of castration is in the air, dance-movement therapists need their strengths in order to neutralize what is happening. A total opening up to the client may indicate great sensitivity and sympathy in the therapist but does not serve clients who need a structure against which to delineate themselves.

An example comes to mind in which a supervisee and her client were so tuned into each other that the therapist felt the client's confusion as her own. She was unable to provide him with a framework for growth because in buying into her client's defensive distortions they could avoid the reality of his stunted life together. She often complained that she could not understand him in the session nor her supervisor in supervision. Confusion reigned. Her sympathy for her client's pathetic helplessness had overwhelmed her own creativity.

Another supervisee also picked up the clues her client gave her but dismissed them as meaningless. In both instances, these therapists were fearful of being swallowed by their clients' needs. Rather than trying to understand what was going on they "sympathized." But because they sympathized and felt sorry for their clients they were unable to empathize. In the first example cited the young therapist was unable to say "no" to her client, who soon led her a merry chase through the halls of the institution where this took place. He wouldn't perform for her at all and regularly showed her his most bizarre behavior. In the second example, a small girl over and over again tried to convey to her therapist that she had been present when her mother gave birth to her brother. The child clutched her abdomen, breathed heavily and loudly, and conveyed pantomimically what she had seen. Her therapist, however, could only see a cute little girl acting in a bizarre manner.

Empathy and understanding was clearly lacking because of strong countertransferential feelings in both therapists. Their countertransferential echoes had not been sufficiently filtered through these therapists' egos, indeed, their own conflicts blinded them.

Sympathy is the first step toward knowing about another person. It prepares the groundwork, so to speak for understanding. In sympathy, however, it is easy to feel: I am above all this. I feel sorry for that person over there. This can appear like a form of patronage to the receiver who might say: You've got some nerve being sorry for me. What makes you think you're in a better position than I?

After having sympathy for one's clients, it is necessary to step out of that role and to leave one' own feelings behind in order to receive fully what the other communicates.

Roy Schafer (1959) defines empathy as "the inner experience of sharing in and comprehending the momentary psychological state of another person"(p. 345). It is similar to the aesthetic experience (Kris, 1952) in that there is no uncontrollable call to action or participation as a means of discharging one's own tensions as there would be in sympathetic mourning or anger. There is no pressing urge to do something immediately to, for, or with the other person. It is, rather, a reflective state of the mind in which the other's feeling state is momentarily felt as one's own, while yet being aware that it is not one' own. At its most fruitful, the empathizer remains removed from, but not above his or her observations, he or she is free to follow upon perception with action or not, without tension or hastiness. An harmonious flow of inner and outer awareness combines to free the empathetic therapist to choose the correct course of intervention without haste or personal need for gratification. Thus the fruit of empathy may serve action that is other-directed, but never in the service of personal need-gratification.

To achieve the necessary distance from one's own conflicts, personal therapy is an essential phase of training. It provides the therapist with the testing and proving ground on which sympathy and intuition can develop into an empathetic tool for interpersonal therapeutic interaction.

The continuous questioning of her own reactions to any given client is compulsory homework for any therapist who hopes to achieve meaningful results. Just as the developmental level of the clients propels them into specific transferences, the countertransferences evoked by close contact are also specific to developmental levels, which should be those of the client rather than the therapist. The would-be therapist who marches into and through the therapeutic process without conscious reactions is repressed at best, insensitive at worst.

Overreactions in the form of needing continuously to talk about one's work on a specific patient are usually indications that clarification either in the form of supervision or through more personal therapy are needed. The key word here is "continuously"—indicating obsessive, helpless rumination without problem-solving. It is desirable to compare notes with colleagues and to seek further information from supervisors and teachers.

REACTIONS TO AUTISM

The autistic client can set off a host of feelings in the therapist. But if anger or disappointment are activitated by the client's refusal to respond, this is not necessarily a bad sign. It could merely be a reflective echo of the client's extreme disorganization and indicate the first glimmer of a relationship. After all, one doesn't get angry at a wall! Anger indicates that the therapist believes the client is withholding something in the way of a workable handle. Boredom is an indication of total lack of success. Both client and therapist feel they would like to do something else but they don't know what. Boredom binds them into a therapeutic stalemate. "Liking" a client despite runny nose, dirty clothes, and unruly behavior is also often a signal that the therapist's unconscious receptors have been at work. It is extremely important in that case to differentiate *what* it is that appeals—does the therapist unconsciously identify with the dirty unruliness, perhaps even admire it because she herself had always been "good"? If such is the case, it would be better to assign the client to someone else, since an unresolved conflict around dirt and messiness would propel the therapist into inappropriate intervention, even though the sessions would feel "good" and "successful" to her, since the client would be acting out the therapist's own repressed impulses. One talented intern allowed a very decompensated, chronically schizophrenic girl whom she liked a lot to peek into the top of her own tights to prove that "they could be girls together who had good vaginas.'' While the overall interpretation had been correct, the intern could not, due to some unresolved conflicts around body-image and sexuality of her own, tolerate nor understand her client's inability to internalize.

The raw, unneutralized drives of psychotics hook like magnets into the unprobed or shaky areas of the therapist's psyche and can only be neutralized by either verbal or nonverbal interpretation. The intern mentioned above would have been better off had she brought pictures or books such as the *Time-Life* series *How Babies Are Made.* She could then have put distance between her raw impulse and actually acting out for her client and herself.

Since autism and the schizophrenias are caused by fixation in, or regression to, the oral stage, countertransferences also bear an oral stamp.

COUNTERTRANSFERENTIAL ORALITY

Therapists confronted by the oral need and greediness of schizophrenic clients may find themselves nauseated or dizzy. The prize for "tuning in" is often the experiencing of part of the client's disorientation. Desirably, this is merely a trial action for the therapist who can come out of such counteridentification with a new understanding of how to reach the client. Balancing and centering exercises are specifics for dizziness, deep inhalations a countering of nausea.

The reasonably well-trained therapist will soon recognize her personal signal indicating that she is about to enter a symbiosis with a client. The becoming-one without boundaries on the oral level is like a mutual swallowing of each other, a giving in, symbolically, to oral-incorporative needs. Again the therapist may experience nausea, a need to eat or drink, or smoke more than normally, or suddenly become superaware of one or another body part. All this gives way to a kind of euphoria when the symbiosis is in its positive stages, so that outrageous demands by the client are met with empathy and

even appear logical when contrasted with his former depriva-
tion. The therapist may even allow herself to share in the patient's omnipotent fantasies of immediate success and total need
gratification if she is not aware of this trap. This phase can be
fruitfully used to lead the client into reality-oriented games,
provided the therapist verbalizes the difference between "you"
and "me" appropriately. The therapist who has strong needs
for tactile stimulations and for being a supermother will have
problems ferrying the client into separation-individuation. As
one client summed it up: "I used to think your breasts were as
large as clouds, filled with a thousand gallons of milk, all for
me." It's a loss not only for the patient to give up that kind of
fantasy!

COUNTERTRANSFERENTIAL UNEASE WITH THE BORDERLINE CLIENT

Clients suffering from Borderline Personality Organization also create special countertransferential problems. Because
they vacillate so often from one extreme to the other, they produce unease. Kohut (1971, 1977) and Kernberg (1975, 1976)
speak of the special countertransferential pull from such clients.
Their wounded narcissism cries out for help so convincingly
and, at certain times, their idolizations of their therapists are so
great, that it is hard for the therapist to remain objective.
Borderline clients feel entitled to special treatment and dispensations due to their sufferings. Kernberg finds that looking inside of himself in response to such clients gives him the clue
about what needs to be pulled into consciousness before the
client verbalizes it. The supposition is that in the Boderline Personality the inner structure is still so shaky that transference
phenomena especially tend to be misused and misrepresented.
Therefore, Kernberg finds his own tuning-in process a more
reliable guide to what's actually going on in the treatment than
the client's productions. Searles (1968) and LeBoit (1979) corroborate the need for such intuitive and empathetic work. They
stress as paramount the therapist's self-knowledge.But self-

knowledge does not necessarily make it easier to hold still when the client idealizes the therapist. After all, self-knowledge is supposed to include knowing that one is not perfect. But accepting the client's view that the therapist is simply and perfectly wonderful is essential. Destroying that view prematurely would destroy the client (Kohut, 1977).

ANALITY AND COUNTERTRANSFERENCE

Once the loss and normal frustration of the oral period have been successfully overcome, there exists prototype experience for dealing with adverse events. Nevertheless, it is often a shock to come into touch with the cold rages and manipulative behavior of the anal-sadistic phase. No matter how aware the therapist is of the defensive nature of many of the ambivalences, it is easy to rear up in anger or to retaliate in kind when the patient provokes and withholds for session after session.

The therapist may find herself reliving old tension patterns, and start to struggle with aggression against the self rather than deal with the client's hostility. Therapists who need to see themselves as good and giving may not be able to confront patients interpretively with their own behavior. Clients who repeatedly swing their fists against the world need a symbolic target and permission to see the therapist as less than perfect. They need to experience the result of the reality their psychic needs set up: If they behave hatefully they will not be loved, not is it the therapist's job to love them. If clients have everything in therapy, why should they try to find anything in their real life? Overindulgence produces pathology both in life and in therapy (Spitz, 1965).

The other side of the coin is represented in the period when obsessional clients have a respite from the compulsions plaguing them and their body is functioning with less restriction but has not yet worked through all the implications of a new state of being-in-the-world. Where they previously could find no positive contact-making device, and couched everything in negative or ambivalent terms, they suddenly, and for a brief time, discover that the therapist can do no wrong. Since this kind of adulation strikes a false note and fairly reeks of manipulation, the therapist usually has a difficult time accepting it. When the patient assures her of her beauty and grace, she suddenly feels ugly and clumsy. When the client declares unremitting love, she finds she needs to go to the toilet. Her unconscious understands fully that the adoration is insincere and has nothing to do with the mature capacity to love. Beginnning therapists often are so startled by this dichotomy between their conscious and unconscious perceptions that they become temporarily blocked in the creation of nonverbal and verbal interpretations, just as the client is still blocked and psychically constipated.

In this event, it is fruitful to institute simple isometric exercises to reassure both client and therapist that the murderous rage soon to explode will annihilate neither one of them.

Therapists feel for and about their clients what the client unconsciously presents them with. But alongside of these manifestations which have their playground in the psychological interior of therapist and client, there is also the real relationship which springs up in therapy as in any other human relationship. For me, its almost impossible not to like and respect another human being I have worked with for some time. I would feel cheated if I did not allow myself to acknowledge this. However, I have learned to keep this "liking" at the background of our interaction so that it does not interfere with the development of transference-countertransference duality of treatment.

Chapter 4

THEORY IN ACTION: THE EGO-PSYCHOANALYTIC APPROACH IN DANCE-MOVEMENT THERAPY APPLIED

In the preceding chapter a developmental focus has been adhered to. The same structure will be followed here, because vestiges of the developmental phases we pass through stay with us throughout life and may surface during times of stress, as has been shown in the chapter on Theory.

Despite the fact that people who are stuck in the oral phase have fewer internal adaptations at their command, therapeutic interaction with them is extraordinarly complex. The therapist has to try to bring order to a universe that is fragmented into many shreds of misperceived experience. Sometimes, this ordering is only temporary and disintegrates again under the blows of external or internal difficulties. The further up the developmental ladder a person has climbed, the less likely he or she is to succumb when adversity strikes. This is apparent when one looks at the cases presented here. There is a wide span, for instance, between Carrie's autistic partial interpersonal relationships and unmodulated perceptions and Raymond's bitterly sardonic view of significant others and the world.

A narrative describing group work with deeply regressed

individuals is included because the actual work is of interest even without the developmental framework. It affords a glimpse at what is possible when working in the adjunctive mode. Clearly it is valuable work which establishes a baseline for further therapeutic intervention. The limitations of the adjunctive mode become equally clear when one compares it to the more fully conceptualized individual case studies.

THE DEVELOPMENT OF AFFECT IN SIX CATATONIC TEENAGERS

During the first meeting, a collective barricade of depressive withdrawal raised itself so impermeably in all six youngsters that the therapist's response was a longing for flight from such helplessness.

Derealization and depersonalization had taken their toll to such an extent that the youngsters seemed to stare blankly out of the prison of their bodies without being able to make more than the most primitive use of their physical equipment.

Chronologically the oldest in a school for emotionally disturbed children, they had one conspicuous feature in common: while some of their ego functions continued to grow within the conflict-free sphere of the ego, as expounded by Hartmann (1958), other development not only stopped but was defended against by further regression at the onset of puberty.

Deneutralized energy appeared to have been turned against the self in an unsuccessful attempt to ward off the demands of an archaic superego, thereby destroying even the last vestiges of object- and self representations. Or, in Jacobson's (1964) terms, there seemed to have taken place a "decrease in the cathexis of the periphery, or perceptive and motor functions, resulting in the cathexis of the body organs with concomitant drive diffusion to the point of prevalence of destructive drive energy which again must be discharged through the physiologic channels in the body"(p. 17).

Schur (1953) speaks of the turning away or attempting to avoid an unfamiliar object by the infant as the first manifestation of an intrapsychic attempt at defense in response to an awareness of discomfort. However, not even this eight-month level of awareness could be ascribed to these youngsters.

Spitz (1965) also describes the eight months' anxiety of the infant when it demands to be with familiar objects and shows displeasure at the intrusion of the unfamiliar.

The egos exhibited in this group had taken the path into extreme sensorimotor inhibitions strongly visible in the musculature. In an attempt to defend against further disintegration they had fallen back on incredibly early psychic structures which allowed for functioning and tension discharge on a very primitive level only.

Dom was the best co-ordinated, and in touch with at least some wedge of reality. Diagnosed as chronically schizophrenic at age six, he became violent when he reached puberty. After a series of six electroshock treatments he had become quiet and withdrawn and now behaved with an affectless docility that was betrayed only by his depressed, bent-kneed, old man's walk. Dom is the second of three children. His family did not avail themselves of the family-therapy sessions offered by the school.

His "special friend" was Sarah, a pretty fourteen year-old whose chronic schizophrenia forced her into a bizarre, physically symbiotic mode of relating (Hartmann, 1958; Rubinfine, 1962; Mahler, 1969). After staring through the therapist, she stalked over on long legs that seemed to be constructed without knees and leaned against her. After she felt the warmth of the therapist's body, she quickly sniffed for some special odor and withdrew back to her place next to Dom. Leaning against people appeared to be her way of making sure they existed, smelling their emanations a way of identifying them. It could be hypothesized that Sarah was at least thermally aware of her mother in early infancy and that she was now constantly in search of the gratification the perception of this odor-warmth had given her. However, Sarah's actions were devoid of affect even during the investigative stage of her behavior.

Sarah's mother reported her development as normal to age two, when she began to withdraw after the parent's separation following violent quarrels which she is said to have witnessed. Sarah is the only child. Her mother attended the school's group sessions regularly but is said to have been extremely resistant. Sarah's diagnosis was made at a local rehabilitation center.

David's diagnostic report labeled him as "schizophrenic with autistic features and retarded." He, too, stared through the therapist then shifted his gaze to a spot on the wall in back of her and began to suck his thumb. Instead of speaking, he often bleated and snorted and tried to bite people. His teachers and parents had tried to train him out of this by not responding to it. He shared the old man's walk with Dom and in addition carried himself with bent shoulders and head.

David indulged in hunger strikes, between ages four and five. He was not toilet-trained until age six. At fourteen, he began to attack his mother and father. He was medicated and consequently calmed down.

The family stopped coming to therapy sessions when the group therapist suggested that David should no longer sleep with his father, a habit he had followed since early childhood. David is the only child.

Fred, fourteen, and Martha, sixteen were also "special friends." Martha's fat abdomen and stiff knees made it hard for her to move efficiently. Nevertheless, she likes to "twist" when she heard music and to hold hands with Fred while she slowly shuffled along in imitation of a dance. At the onset of her psychosis at age eight, she had been in treatment with a psychoanalytically-oriented psychotherapist. Treatment was discontinued by her parents when it became apparent that Martha's illness prevented her from taking in and learning and that would have to be placed in a special school. Her parents first reported to have noticed something different when Martha was five and often would not speak. Martha smiled at the therapist that first session, but made sure that there was no eye contact.

Fred was the activist of the group. Winding himself up, babbling incoherently, he would suddenly jump up and spin like a top. His greeting was a spinning, spinning closer to the therapist, coming to a halt, and then walking away from her decisively. His spinning was understood as autoerotic tension release. The others in the group watched Fred seriously. His behavior appeared to have some special meaning for them that aroused at least momentary interest.

Fred was diagnosed as "schizophrenic with autistic features" at age four. His parents took him to a local mental health center because of continuous head-banging and echolalia. He received psychoanalytically-oriented psychotherapy until age twelve when he began to regress and to hallucinate. Residential treatment was suggested but the parents "could not bear to give him up."

Fred is the third of three children. His parents attended the family therapy sessions regularly until the father has a car accident in which he injured his head. The father began to fear for his sanity, and began to brood, refusing all offered help. Fred's catatonic phase started approximately at the time of his father's injury.

Mary, fifteen, had rescued herself from the disequilibrium of a boundary-less world by becoming a robot. The grimace of a smile pasted on her face, she would wipe the same spot for an hour or sweep the floor over and over until someone stopped her. Despite her diagnosis of both schizophrenia and retardation she was able to put together complicated puzzles and to do petit point embroidery. She walked stiff-kneed, swaying a little from side to side, arms bent upward at the elbows, wrists limp, hands dangling. Her unawareness of the therapist's presence seemed less defensive than that of some of the others. She did not even find it necessary *not* to see the therapist. The second of two children, she came from a broken home and is said to have been physically abused by her stepfather until that marriage, too, was dissolved.

The intial diagnosis of four of the youngsters were made by neurologists and only later confirmed by diagnostic evaluations of psychiatric teams, two at State Mental Hospital, two at local Rehabilitation Centers. The other youngsters were diagnosed at local Mental Health Clinics. Psychoanalytically-oriented therapies were not recommended for any of them after their most recent evaluation.

The assignment to "do something" with this group placed the therapist in the position of having to offer herself as a possibly significant person to very regressed young people. Their psychic immobilization was part of the defense against recognition of their own inability to reach out for gratification. This was also the suppression of all desire to be taken care of by some other-than-self; i.e., part object relationships had to be abandoned because the anxiety aroused by either imagined or real, internal and/or external stimulation was so extreme that the budding ego had become paralyzed in its efforts to cope with the act of living and developing. This left the youngsters prey to the repetitious cycle of erupting drives and their control by whatever poorly designed measure of their hard-pressed organisms.

To make pleasure available once more, to offer another chance at the felt experience of living growth, to encourage the development of affect out of the dense burden of undifferentiated anxiety, whichever way one could phrase it, there was no obvious approach discernible.

In these six youngsters the freezing of affect states and loss of inner body sensitivities had occurred to an amazing degree. In order to preserve themselves from utter self-destruction they had chosen to become literally stiff. Therefore, the therapeutic approach had to concern itself directly with an attempt to loosen the youngsters' physical rigidity and to approach those parts of their fragmented egos still accessible to stimuli. To make movement per se a desirable activity once more, to activate immobilized ego functions rather than to allow further petrification of both psyche and soma, were the tasks at hand.

Looking for an approach, the therapist began to examine the reactions she had received.

Fred's response to his perception of an other-than-self, the therapist, had been of interest to his companions, constituting perhaps a fleeting, not quite conscious and therefore not yet usable memory trace of activity as self-gratification. The therapist decided to imitate his spin in the center of the room, saying, "This is the way Fred spins." Mary batted her eyelids rapidly. "Mary shows me; yes, this is the way Fred spins," the therapist interpreted. "Herman's Hermits are heard hissing," Fred answered, with an engaging grin.

Instead of a verbal interpretation the therapist put on a rock and roll record and began to dance a simple back and forth rock step with bent knees, loose arms, and nodding head, because Herman's Hermits were a rock group then in vogue.

Martha immediately got up and did her "twist," an inept, semicircular movement of her hips. Sarah hopped from one foot to another with Dom. Fred danced an acceptable version of a rock dance, talking to an imaginary partner. Mary turned her face to the wall and David started to bleat.

To help him abreact his tension in a more productive way, the therapist showed David how to stamp his feet rhythmically in time to the music, hoping that the repetitive beat would give him comfort as well as a chance to feel his legs in action against the supporting floor. He placed his hands over his ears but tried to mimic the therapist. The rhythm eluded him. The therapist stood close to him, so close that he had to feel her legs move against his side. For a second, he bleated in terror but then relaxed enough to pick up the beat from her movement. When the record ended, he snarled and threatened to bite.

His displeasure was interpreted verbally as an attempt to keep the music going. He was shown how to work the record player so he could provide himself with music. But he had decided that the therapist was the magic music-maker and declined to learn. His previous attempts at self-gratification must have been so disastrous that instead of favoring growth they had confirmed for him the terrors of a universe in which no helpful, need-ministering other-than-self existed. But he did allow the therapist to show him a new discharge pattern, the rhythmic stamping, which had given him enough pleasure to wish for its continuance. It was hoped that eventually it would be possible to enlarge on this primitive basis, so that David's diffuse and agressive behavior could perhaps become tempered.

Margaret Mahler (1967) stresses that autonomous ego development and socially adaptive behavior will not emerge unlees the object-mother is libidinally available. Since David had at least partially responded to mothering attempts the therapist allowed herself to be hopeful.

The contents of the entire first session was encouraging. The traces of conscious perception, almost forming part object relations visible in Sarah's behavior, Dom's depressive walk either as defense against intrusion of the real object world or as the illustration of an introjected object, Fred's ability to make his needs known, and David's willingness to accept body contact and to learn from it, all pointed toward the need for a structured, safe environment where taking-in and the reintegration of disavowed body parts and feelings could take place.

The collective response to rhythmic sound has also been good. All the youngsters had shown the ability to translate heard sound into a physical response activity, even if, as in Mary's turning away, it was no more than a denial.

Each youngster had also been asked simply to walk across the room. Not one of them was able to do so with natural coordination. Their legs and feet were generally turned out, adversely effecting their equilibrium. The knees were also used improperly, either forced into a permanent bend as with Dom and David, or made entirely useless by rigid locking.

The next few months were spent trying to rediscover the dimensions of space in relationship to the body, in finding possibilities for encouraging kinetic awareness, and in attempts to form a workable body image.

Since everybody was stimulated by rock and roll music, each session was started by dancing to it.

The youngsters were encouraged to look at and to imitate the therapist, starting with a vigorous nodding "yes," then shoulder-shaking, then lifting one shoulder at a time; next, elbows were touched with hands, wrists were shaken in the air, and so on, until each part had been in motion.

It was hoped that the vigor of the proposed exercises would

reach into the petrified and distorted equilibrium of the youngsters and charge them with sufficient neutralized energy to "look and listen" to a possible libidinal object, the therapist, once more.

The group was positioned in a circle facing inward when this series of uncomplicated movements was introduced. Therapist, the teacher, and aide participated.

The aim was to block out possible distraction from outside the circle and to foster the perception of the therapist as a leader whom it was safe to follow, someone who might just possibly provide some gratification, and thus stimulate eagerness and fascination with the environment such as the infant experiences when there is an awareness that gratification is associated with activity.

Fortunately the teacher and the aide enjoyed both the music and the simple choreography.

The youngsters watched stupefied during the first demonstration until Martha saved the day. "Yes, yes," she said, and nodded her head stiffly. "Yes, yes," said Dom, Fred, and Sarah, but didn't move their heads. David began to bob his torso up and down, Mary smiled widely. "Everybody says yes," the therapist interpreted, and beamed approval as strongly as she could.

On repeating the whole series of movement it was noticed that all the youngsters tightened their neck tendons to such an extent that the area around the mouth became unduly rigid, making the simple act of nodding the head an intricate and possibly painful maneuver.

Martha must have been full of good will to give a nodded "yes" when her involuntary muscular response so obviously was a danger signal. The locked jaws and the desperate thrust to achieve control certainly looked more like an attempt to keep out poison than to learn. Yet they were all willing to try. Maybe some of the therapist's urgency had reached them enough to want something for themselves again, the something being either food or mother, or both, since the tensions were most visible around the mouth. Food, after all, initially comes from others at a time when perceptions are still immature.

Awareness of the head as the seat of much of the sensory apparatus prompted the therapist to seek for a way to address that body part directly. Everyone was asked to sit comfortably on the floor and a hypnotically slow and soft record was played. The therapist demonstrated a slow, steady head roll.

The group responded astonishingly well. There were not habitual headrollers among the youngsters. Yet everyone seemed to understand the value of relaxing and rolling. Everyone, that is, but Fred.

"It's going to fall off," he wailed, holding his head up stiffer and higher than ever. Seeing the panic rise in his eyes, the therapist placed her hand firmly on his head and looked at him.

"This is your head. It belongs to you," she informed him. He put his hand on her head and began to feel and press it until he had satisfied himself that the therapist possessed a head which would fall off her shoulders. Apparently reassured, he stopped moaning.

Fred and the therapist were to go through these castration anxieties many times. It was always the fact that the therapist's head would not fall off, both symbolically, by not being frightened, and actually, that reassured Fred and paved the way toward his liking the therapist's head. A part object relationship began to form.

Much later it was discovered that Fred had introjected part of his mother's attitude toward himself. In a paroxysm of self-punishment and fear, he had used the symptom of the falling head to express both his wish and his fear that his mother's standard sayings, "I'm going to lose my mind if you keep annoying me," and "You're giving me a splitting headache," might become reality.

In tactilely experiencing the firmness of the therapist's head and neck, Fred allowed a small particle of reality to illuminate and restructure part of his ego. He perceived enough reality to make a connection with his own confused thought processes so that verbalization rather than somatization became possible.

In the meantime the rest of the group were still rolling their heads in perfect contentment. They fell into a state resembling the comfortable bliss just before sleep. Not quite knowing whether much needed gratification had been provided or just another avenue for withdrawal, the therapist said goodbye to each youngster individually, stating which day she would be back for the next session.

The therapist formulated at this point that it should be possible to supply and stir the demand for "kernels of early infantile self-images that are the memory traces of pleasurable and unpleasurable sensations, which under the influence of autoerotic and of beginning functional activities and of playful general body investigation became associated with body image"(Jacobson, 1964, p. 20).

The teacher was asked to do something nodding with the group in order to provide the youngsters daily with at least a threshold experience. She reported when the therapist returned that everyone, including Fred, had been willing. Only David was still unable to nod, and bent his entire torso instead. Apparently he had to defend himself even more rigidly against feeling anything in the mouth region because of his strong, often, acted-out oral incorporative needs. The fusion of head, torso, and neck seemed to provide the muscular defense against the urge to bite and destroy.

The sessions stayed on a pretty even level for some weeks with the youngsters learning to function more efficiently and taking pleasure in this, concluding with either headrolls or deep-breathing exercises. Although they knew the therapist by name and smiled when she appeared, David and Fred had been the only ones who had allowed her to help them individually. No group feeling of any kind had emerged yet. Fred still regularly spun away as a greeting; David bleated and couldn't nod; Mary mainly ignored the proceedings and stood in the circle; in short, another way of reaching this largely nonverbal group had to be found.

The slightly better muscular functioning seemed to occur only during the sessions themselves. No difference of any sort was reported by either teachers or parents in the somnambulic path these youngsters traced through their days.

The next approach was based on the assumption that the previous attempts at body image building had been only partially successful because it had not reached the group at their psychic age level.

Twelve month-old babies like to reach up, stand on tiptoe, reach for mother's hand, etc. So that would have to be the psychomotor level one would have to try for, something not too hard kinesthetically, but beyond the body image and object relations formation of most people in the group.

Once again a circle on the floor was used. To smooth waltz music arms were lifted above the head, then spread to the side. The "up" action of the arms was familiar to all but all stopped raising them somewhere at the level of the ears. When alternating arms, most would only raise them to the level of the shoulders, or merely bend the elbows in recognition of instruction. Dom, with an agonized look, sometimes managed to raise his arms all the way, but always let them drop at the earliest possible moment.

Suggestions to look at the arms while raising them was met by withdrawal and confusion.

Too much had been demanded. Looking even at one's own, or perhaps particularly at one's own body was a dangerous action, the space above the head enemy territory that might or might not belong to oneself, just as the hand or head might or might not belong to oneself, and might be either animate or inanimate.

The therapist now devised a game to be played daily, called "This is my head." Seated in a circle, the teacher or aide would call out the sentence and as the youngsters chose to comply or not, would place themselves opposite the people who had achieved the action. Then they would say "This is your head. It is a nice head. It is yours," as approvingly as possible. On the days that everyone was "with it" the game would include "Put your hand on my head."

At first, there was much straining and tension and shying away from touching and possible destroying or not finding one's own head or that of the instructor's. But with repeated success and volumes of praise the youngsters viewed the game as just that, an activity that was enjoyed, giggled at, and looked forward to, in exactly the way babies reach with much concentration for an object, relax on finding it, and eventually just rely on the integrated cathected memory of the action to repeat it.

They had by now experienced the fact that their heads sat firmly on their shoulders, had learned to gratify themselves to a small degree by testing part of their own physical reality, but what about the reaching up and out?

Once again the therapist decided to play the part of the benevolent but intrusive mother.

With everyone sitting on the floor, she went from one to the next and asked them to look at her. As their faces turned to her in apprehension and awe, she demanded even more. "Touch my head," she asked, bending down only far enough for them barely to reach. Dom and Sarah were the first to comply. Dom seemed horribly worried at his own aggression. The therapist smiled and pulled him up. The waltzes usually played during games were turned on. The therapist fell into a simple step which Dom picked up immediately. He lost his frown and began to smile. They waltzed till the very end of a long-playing record. Dom's expression changed from worried, to placid, to dreamy, to preoccupied. When the music ended, he seemed startled and held on to the therapist for a little while to reorient himself.

During the time the music was playing he had indeed allowed himself to merge with the therapist's movements and the rhythm of the music, perhaps preparing the ground once more for the beginning of a symbiosis. After this experience he became noticeably attached to the therapist and eager to please her. Teachers and parents were still met with his customary affectless docility.

Sarah reached up eagerly. She was cuddled and smiled at

while she exhibited the behavior of a happy baby playing with her mother.

Mary went through the motion of reaching up and finding the therapist's head, but with closed eyes. Making contact was too difficult yet, as was completely refusing.

David became more and more hostile as his turns approached each time. After about 3 months he could not control his excitation any longer. He jumped up and bit the therapist hard in the shoulder. "Ouch," she yelled. He giggled, slapped his thigh, pointed at her. After all the years of having his "naughty" behavior ignored, somebody finally acknowledged it. His bliss knew no bounds. It was as though the recognition of his bite were also the recognition of his own existence.

"I know you would like to eat me all up," the therapist finally managed to interpret. More confirmative glee. Finally, he hugged the therapist and put his head on her shoulder. Shortly after this, he tried to bite his teacher also. Taking her clue from the therapist, she conveyed that she understood and had no difficulty with him after that. Later, he turned the same hostile symptom against himself in order to preserve his hard-won relationships with his teacher and therapist.

The general atmosphere in the group gradually began to change at this point. There seemed to be more willingness to try new things. Withdrawal, a favorite defense with all of them, occurred less frequently in the therapist's presence and the first dawning of object relationships became discernible in everyone. Along with this a definite change in body stance and gait took place.

Sarah and Martha began to use their knees while walking and Dom tried to stand up straight. Natural oppositional swing of arms and legs while walking was still missing. However, teachers and aides reported that the therapist had been asked for by name in between sessions and that music and records had become favorite free-time occupations.

Conspicuously lacking also was any kind of awareness of each other except where special attachments were formed as a rather masturbatory mirror image as with Dom and Sarah. They somehow managed to hop from one foot to another repetitively, hopelessly locked in a mutual haze of dedifferentiation.

From exploring the space above the head, the group now moved to measuring the area immediately to the side of the body again. Arms were opened and gathered in, hugging the torso close. Waltzes were employed as rhythm-makers again as the group sat in a circle on the floor. What a surprise, people bumped into each other! Eyes tried to read the therapist's. What do you do when you touch another's shoulder and chest? The therapist was careful *not* to give a clue. The time had come for less direction. Mary and Sarah were the only ones totally unaffected by feeling the physical presence of their neighbors. They just kept moving and sat staring into space.

Fred finally muttered accusingly: "She's there. My arm is there." "Martha sits next to you," the therapist answered.

Both Martha and Fred became excited. They turned to each other and giggled. They spread out their arms, but, having turned to face each other rather than the circle, didn't touch. Finally, Fred carefully placed his hand on Martha's shoulder. Together, they turned back to the circle.

When the exercises were resumed the therapist placed her hand on her neighbor's shoulders and imitated Fred. Startled, Dom and Sarah looked at her. She smiled and gave verbal explanations. Now Dom decided he could be aggressive too, and placed his hand on the therapist's shoulder. Somehow, this was funny and mirth spread all around the circle. Yes, we were really all there, sitting on the floor with our arms on each other's shoulders. The therapist leaned first toward Dom, then toward Sarah. Slowly, and at first raggedly, the entire circle followed again giggling and laughing, sometimes experimentally pulling harder to one side than to the other, but in time to the music.

Finally, all were swaying together, happily rocking each other. All relaxed together without anyone finding it necessary to disappear into their private world.

The next time the therapist arrived, everybody immediately positioned themselves on the floor and placed their arms on each other's shoulders.

A way had been found to give each other what each lacked, the comfort and warmth of rocking and being rocked as an infant is rocked and merges both with the act and the person who takes care of him, until the memory of the gratifying experience is cathected and permits, on the earliest level of development, hallucination of gratification until the environment once again actually responds to the expressed need.

Mary still seemed untouched. Drawn into the circle by the others, she now opened her eyes but stayed as far away from the therapist as possible. However, the staying away had a defensive quality, quite different from the genuinely unseeing stare she had initially used.

The youngsters now began to sway and dance in the therapist's absence too, and tried to explore the physical presence of teachers and aides and parents and each other by touching and hugging. The parents were startled by this new approach behavior and feared a turn for the worse, but allowed themselves to be reassured by the staff.

During the next phase of doing sit-ups and bicycling exercises with the legs, Mary happened to be next to the therapist. She couldn't even bend and stretch her legs together, let alone pump them separately in a bicycling fashion. The therapist bent over her and asked her to place her feet flat against her chest and to push the therapist up, the kind of fun and nonsense one does while diapering a baby. Looking puzzled, she gave a tentative push, then another one. It worked. Her pat grimace dissolved into a real smile. Then the group called the therapist back volubly. What did she mean, playing with Mary so long, Fred wanted to know. Sibling rivalry was beginning to rear its head! What a long, long way from the silent autoerotic headrolling of previous sessions!

From this point onward, work with the group moved along less arduous channels. The more often they moved actively in relation to the therapist, the more clearly feelings of bliss, fear, and trust began to emerge.

Many specific, analyzable fantasies came to the surface and some memories were verbally expressed instead of being acted out and illustrated in symptoms.

Withdrawal as a defense against the taking-in process became much less pronounced, and attention spans became more nearly normal.

Collectively, an atmosphere of expectation and a greater willingness to relate to each other arose.

While much work still remained to be done, every youngster in the group had shown much improvement both psychically and physically after a period of 9 months.

Shifting the initial therapeutic goal from probing for psychic conflict to an attempt at rebuilding the damaged body image through exercise and dance allowed for approach techniques which deal directly with the physical functioning of the body self, thus reducing tension through the utilization of those ego apparati still contained within the conflict-free sphere of the ego. Self and part object representations were seen to form slowly after muscular functioning became less diffuse, and more goal-directed.

In general, the success of object-related sensorimotor activity seemed to foster a tendency toward internalization of both the gratifying activity and the formation of a more adequate body image, leading in turn to renewed attempts at intrapsychic differentiation of the self and other-than-self.

CASE HISTORIES

Dance-Movement Therapy as a Primary Therapy

During the early years as a primary therapist, this writer's caseload consisted primarily of individuals who had been seen by many other kinds of therapists. Dance-Movement therapy was the last resort for families whose hopes had been raised and shattered repeatedly. They tended to hand over their afflicted family member with a combination of resignation, shame, fury, and carefully concealed hope that was often reproduced in the sessions by the client. It was always requested that the family seek help also. A list of colleagues to choose from was supplied. In the beginning this writer saw primarily children who needed to "own" her completely and could not tolerate any but superficial contact with their parents. Nevertheless, the treatment plan always included reintegration of the stricken member in the family structure. Sometimes children whose families were not willing to investigate their own needs were taken on. The results were always curtailed. Children cannot change their own worlds as an adult can. They simply do not have the power to do so. Therefore, families must be involved. In cases where families are too burned out or conflicted to accept offered help, one must accept the limitations which automatically result. Economic realities were always taken into consideration. Families were referred to clinics and clinicians whose fees were compatible with incomes.

The art of successful referring warrants a book by itself. Some people clearly want nothing to do with therapists of any sort.

It isn't always easy to stay emotionally available to someone whose message is a consistent "Go away." Nevertheless, once a family or individual arrives at a therapist's doorstep, this can be a sign that they want to make use of what is offered despite all their disavowals. My personal tenacity springs less from any therapeutic optimism than from an unending fascination with people and their individual ways of being in the world.

The case histories detailing such individual ways follow.

***

From Secondary Autism to Symbiosis

Carrie

Although the prognosis in correctly diagnosed cases of autism is poor, sometimes it is possible to establish "a working alliance" (Friedman, 1969) of a primitive nature by addressing the therapeutic effort to the intact ego apparatus (Hartmann, 1958) and by focusing both verbal and nonverbal interpretations on concrete realities.

In the report presented here, a nonverbal girl took the step from secondary autism to symbiosis during the third year of her therapy.

Carrie was referred at age three and a half by her mother's therapist. The mother had sought professional help when a long string of specialists concurred that Carrie was emotionally disturbed, had a developmental lag, suffered from a possible neurological deficit, and was retarded or autistic or both. The mother could no longer cope with the anxiety engendered by the differing diagnoses and apparently hoped that her own therapy would teach her how to cope with the child. The mother's therapist referred Carrie because at that time nobody else had agreed to take on the child for therapeutic intervention, and residential treatment appeared to be the only remaining option.

Presenting symtoms were: (1) lack of speech; she had a vocabulary of two words, "Ma," and "No," which were used to express any and everything; (2) hyperactivity with varied periods of catatonic rigidity, in which Carrie would stand on tiptoe with one arm raised above her head and stare into space; (3) toe-walking; (4) lip-smacking, and (5) a peculiar shaking of the hands.

On reading the reports by the speech therapist, the psychiatrist, and neurologist who had seen Carrie, it was easy to become confused, because there simply was a lack of cohesion among the diagnosis. I agreed to see the child together with her mother to form an initial impression. The neurological examination did not include an EEG, because the father put his foot down and decided sharply that there was nothing wrong with Carrie's brain. As it turned out, his insistence reflected good unconscious insight into his daughter's pysche; later on, it was discovered that there was a great deal of body image distortion centered on the head area, and an EEG might have reinforced the fantasies Carrie had about herself.

During the first interview, Carrie's mother was obviously frightened and held herself rigidly erect in her chair. She answered all questions in painstaking detail. Carrie's delivery had been normal, but she had not wanted a child at that time. She added this latter phrase with a guilty look at Carrie, who was standing quietly in the room looking at nothing in particular. Carrie had been an active baby and did not like being held. She ate well, stood at eight months, walked at twelve months. At eighteen months she was hospitalized for 3 days with the croup and was tied down screaming in her crib inside the oxygen tent. At two years of age she had to have her nose cauterized, and this was done in the pediatrician's office with a nurse and the mother holding the screaming Carrie down.

Mrs. A knew from her own therapist that this might have been wrong and broke into an anxiety sweat when she recounted this tale.

She came from a blue-collar family in which there was never "any time for her." She married at twenty-four. Carrie's father was regarded as a good catch, "an engineer employed by the government." His hobby is "looking at stars." At first he was much opposed to his wife's therapy but adjusted to it, because they learned to "talk" to each other.

Mrs. A described Carrie as very attached to her father. He could calm her down when nobody else could.

During this interview Carrie was in the room. A well-stocked bowl of goodies is kept in this writer's studio. Carrie had discovered it. She had taken it from the desk onto the floor, placed it between her legs and was chomping away. She grunted with pleasure and sniffed the treats, unwrapped a lot of it, and made a little pile of the unwrapped and the wrapped pieces, never mixing the two. More than by the ability to differentiate between the two kinds of food, the way she fed herself was significant. She gave herself over to the pleasure of eating completely. She was like a tiger cub with his first hunk of meat.

When Mrs. A became aware of this, she swooped down on Carrie and tried to wrestle the treats away from her. After struggling silently for a while with Carrie snatching what she could and Mrs. A grabbing away what she could, she burst into tears and said, "I don't want to give her up. But I can do nothing with her."

After the second interview, Mrs. A's therapist called up and asked what had gone on. Mrs. A was reluctant to place Carrie in therapy with this therapist because she was afraid Carrie would be indulged too much. At this point no statement had been made either way about my readiness to take Carrie on.

The affect Carrie had shown while eating her treats was an encouraging sign. Truly autistic children like to eat candy too, but they do not show the capacity to enjoy themselves as aggressively as Carrie had done. Her ability to differentiate between two types of candy also could be seen as a type of conflict-free sphere in her undeveloped ego. Certainly she could look at something and perceive its differences so that there might be a possibility of working with that particular ego apparatus. Neurological damage would have to be minimal because of her truly amazing facility to unwrap candy quickly and efficiently and then pile it into separate little heaps.

I cautiously agreed to see Carrie for a trial period of 3 months, three times a week. On the first visit, Carrie came into the room willingly enough. She made a beeline for the candy and literally knelt herself into the business of gratifying herself. Music was playing. The therapist tried to coax Carrie into swaying with her. When her hand was touched Carrie pulled back as though she were about to be killed and emitted a sound of such ferocity that it was easy to empathize with the mother. It really would be easy to be intimidated by her. Various other approach techniques were tried, such as gongs and bells which could be struck or rung rhythmically, but there was no response, no matter how much noise was made. This is very atypical for autistic children who usually look up blandly and listen.

Carrie blocked the therapist out completely and intentionally. The therapist sat down and just watched her. It took 2 weeks to find a way to approach her. Whatever was said or done was simply not acknowledged except when the therapist tried to come physically close to Carrie. Then she growled. The therapist finally decided to make some comment about the quality of her chomping because it seemed that she was devouring a universe, rather than just candy. At this time there was no way of knowing whether she could understand anything that was said. All verbal approaches had been ignored. In order not to stir up more id material, the therapist decided to say something that had to do with the here and now. "You have strong teeth," was the comment when Carrie once again gorged herself. She stopped, for the first time, looked at the therapist, and bared her teeth like fangs. "Yes, you do have strong teeth," the therapist repeated without responding to the hostile aspect of her snarl. She started to giggle and ate a little less quickly. She was asked to come to the mirror, which she did willingly. She looked into the mirror and again bared her teeth. The therapist looked on approvingly. When she again began to stuff her mouth, she chewed for a while, then grabbed the therapist's hand and spit the whole mess into it. The therapist said, "You want me to have candy too." This was an incorrect response. In subsequent sessions it developed that the spitting into the therapist's hand had been a symbolic taking possession of the therapist as part object. Carrie did not respond verbally but began to take a cache of candy home with her. It was not possible to ascertain whether this had any symbolic significance and helped to preserve her from possible separation anxiety, or whether it was merely a way of getting more candy easily. Either way, the therapist acquiesced because she felt that any kind of gratification was sorely needed.

Her mother became very upset and began to threaten to

take Carrie out of therapy since she was indulged so much. Fortunately, her own therapist managed to persuade her to stick out at least the 3 months' trial period.

Things now began to happen fast and furiously. Carrie would come in, eat a few pieces of candy and then use the therapist's hand to point to a toy or a thing she wanted. But if the therapist tried to touch her, she still emitted a growl. It was not then entirely clear what this use of the therapist's hand represented, whether it was the beginning of a part object relationship or whether Carrie's self-representations was so hazy that she literally could not tell where she started and the therapist began. However, the way in which she used the hand seemed to indicate that she saw her environment realistically, since she wanted blocks piled up, dolls in her lap, cups on the table. Perhaps using the hand was similiar to the neonate's use of its mother's body rhythms and libidinal availability to learn and absorb. At any rate, with the therapist's hand to protect her from possible danger, she managed to play with toys in a relatively organized way. The therapist always verbalized what they were doing together and made a point of telling her: "This is my hand, this is your hand."

In the meantime, the mother had a great deal to cope with. Apparently Carrie's dawning relationship with her therapist put a kink into her relationship with her mother. (Hartmann, 1950; Jacobson, 1964; Mahler, 1969). On one occasion, they had a minor car accident coming to the session because Mrs. A said she was nervous; another time they arrived an hour early, and Mrs. A repeatedly needed to use the therapist's bathroom. In short, signs that Carrie had permitted her therapist to enter her psychic world, and thus her mother's, multiplied.

Carrie liked the mirror in the studio very much. She would pull the therapist in front of it, and together they would admire her strong teeth until the day came when she reached up and began to examine the therapist's teeth. She giggled and appeared delighted. This was verbalized and she nodded. At this time she stopped using the therapist's hand. Then came a phase of cooking play. She would drag out all the little pots and pans and cook all sorts of things. Her behavior with the candy changed, too. She would put one piece in the garbage can, one piece on the floor, and then cook some for herself before eating. The 3 months were up by this time, and it was decided that Carrie should stay, despite the fact that her eating behavior at home had become horrendous. She had become picky in what she ate. Some of the food had to be on the floor, some in the garbage. By placing her food in different places she seemed to perpetuate the early split between an all-good and an all-bad mother (Spitz, 1965).

Her strong hostility and fantasies of destruction were expressed during the cooking episodes. She would tear some plastic dolls limb from limb and then feed a toy monkey, the open kitchen stove, anything, showing clearly that she was not able to differentiate animate and inanimate objects. Some interpretation of this behavior like "You want the monkey to eat your food, but not the doll," had no effect. However, she did begin to say words. After 6 months she "cooked," and spoke about "meatballs, spaghetti, hot dogs, lollipops," and on one occasion, candy soup for the "candy lady," her spontaneous name for the therapist. She was thanked for the candy soup which she fed the therapist with a spoon. She kept repeating "Good, good." The entire oral-sadistic phase was re-enacted, this time, however, with some attempts within the ego to use partially neutralized energy.

The bizarre behavior of lip-smacking and the motions of the hand disappeared entirely after 9 months, although they had never been specifically dealt with. When the mother was asked about the stiff stance on toes, she realized, with a shock, that Carrie had given that up too.

Some of Carrie's energy must have been neutralized enough at this time to be channeled into the productive and gratifying channel of part object relationships and a corresponding increase of the awareness of self.

She also became willing to play body image games in which she and the therapist sang "Put your hand on your shoulders, knees," etc. She could soon perform this adequately but was unable to touch her head or nose. She often shook her head as though bewildered, hit at the mirror image of her head and in every way showed that she both feared and disliked it.

Her favorite game was still the cooking game, including feeding the therapist. She also began to eye a baby bottle with great interest. Mrs. A. was pregnant again and Carrie picked up a whole new set of words: baby, diaper, bottle, pregnant, milk. When the baby was about to be born, the mother's therapist called and asked that Carrie be prepared for the birth since the mother contemplated putting sour milk into a bottle and giving it to Carrie in an attempt to keep her weaned. Having heard that children sometimes regress at the birth of a sibling, she thought she would break Carrie of it before it happened. Mrs. A.'s therapist had not been able to convince her that tricking Carrie might be harmful. The therapist decided that it might be best to precipitate, just as Mrs. A. wanted to do, but in a different direction.

Ordinarily the therapist would have waited until Carrie had picked up and used a bottle by herself. The therapist decided to show Carrie that it was all right to do it now. It was hoped that it would be possible to contain a regression if Carrie had a chance to work out some of her feeling before the baby was born. The gamble was that there might be traces of gratification available to her by now. During the next session a bottle was filled with water and Carrie was told that babies drink from them. She took the clue with alacrity, carried the bottle around with her, cradled it in her arms as though it were a baby, poured the water out and filled it up again. In short, she did everything but drink from it.

After several sessions of playing around with the bottle, which was always placed prominently in sight filled with water, she finally took it, turned her back to the therapist and tentatively took a swig. Keeping her voice neutral, the therapist said, "You drank out of the bottle," whereupon she threw it into a corner and ran panic-stricken about the room. Wondering what kind of a trauma weaning must have been for her, the therapist picked the bottle up, filled it again and placed it on the table. This time Carrie came up with a different idea. As of old, she took the therapist's hand and placed it on the bottle. She left her hand there but did nothing else. Then Carrie lifted both the bottle and the therapist's hand and placed the nipple in her mouth. The result was interesting. With the sucking she seemed to remember something, some gratifications or warmth—she reached toward the therapist with her other hand and snuggled into her lap with a contented sigh. When she had finished, she said, "Good girl." The therapist repeated, "Good girl." Apparently she had been able to recapture memory traces of gratification, just as had been hoped. The use of the hand had apparently served to protect her from becoming overwhelmed by instinctual needs. Although Carrie did not know enough words to corroborate the therapist's assumption that we had been dealing with a fear of being poisoned and the revengeful wish *to* poison, the sequence of events described lent evidence to the "fear of poison" formulation. Its resolution was visible in the following events.

Drinking out of the bottle now became as important a game as cooking. Sometimes Carrie would fill the bottle, at other times, ask the therapist to do it. When she finally offered to share the bottle with the therapist, she said, "No, grownups and big children prefer to drink out of cups." Carrie poured some water out of the bottle into a toy cup and gave it to the therapist, who drank it and thanked her. One of the hazards of working with children like this consists of possibly having to drink a thousand cups of water. The therapist did, always offering the same explanation, until Carrie finally decided it would be nice if she, too, would drink out of a cup. When she made the decision that it was all right to drink out of a cup, the ritual of throwing some of her food away disappeared, as though it had been the weaning trauma which had made it so difficult for her to accept what was offered. The ritual had been a defense against the strong urge to devour, as well as the fear of being devoured or possibly poisoned.

Mrs. A.'s pregnancy became very visible. Carrie became preoccupied with stomachs, passing gas, and feces, greatly shocking her mother. She began to smear play-dough around the doll's bottom and tried to flush the doll down the toilet. She also began to carry water into the studio and to wash the floor with it. If she spilled water, she would say, "Oh, shit."

She talked a lot to herself. But her mother complained that Carried talked more "for the therapist than for her." Carrie's hyperactivity increased and she became accident-prone, at one time needing stitches in her lip, at another spraining an ankle, etc. Mrs. A. complained that once again she could "do nothing with her." Somehow Carrie tried anything new too energetically, totally devoid of fear, as though her ego could not quite keep up with the task of reality-testing.

During the sessions, however, Carrie's games became more and more coherent. How to give the baby a bath was discussed after she smeared the doll with play-dough; she learned how to dress and undress a doll, and how to diaper it.

She also began to take an interest in puzzles. Here she showed that she still had problems differentiating animate and inanimate by yelling "ouch" every time she stuck a piece of the puzzle in the right place. Sensory stimuli became important, to feel things, pieces of cloth and fur, hot and cold water. An entire educative period ensued in which Carrie learned about her environment by touching and feeling.

When her brother was born, she barely reacted at home but intensified her doll games in sessions.

When the baby was about three months old, an acute depression set in. Carrie began to cry when her father went to work, would periodically stop her games at home and cover her eyes to sob for long periods on end. She would not let her mother console her.

The intrusion of the real world into her till then boundaryless universe, the birth of the sibling, had formed an unbearable loss. Also, the realization that she was at least partially separate from her mother and could not at all control her father were too much for her. Specifically, one day she put a piece of paper between her legs and said, "This is not for little girls, this for mother's blood." How do you explain mensis to a four and a half year old? She was told that mother was not hurt. She answered: "I did it, I did it."

When it was again explained to her that little girls cannot hurt their mothers in that way, that the blood was not her fault, that she had not killed mother, she again sobbed, "I did, I did."

After several sessions of this, she began to make boys out of play-dough with gigantic penises and informed the therapist that she "wanted to make boys." This was the first step in her identification with mother. It was also discussed that boys indeed have penises and girls, vaginas. All discussions were deliberately kept on a reality level. Her behavior was not interpreted as a wish for a penis because it was feared that Carrie's ego could not acknowledge and integrate the wishes of her id.

Her whole behavior pattern began to change at this time, indicating a shift caused by castration anxiety. She became quiet and subdued and took to bathing the doll in a gentle soothing manner, showing a great deal of tension and apprehension. During the monthly interview with her mother, Mrs. A. reported that Carrie was "good as gold," talked a lot and played "nice and quiet." The change appeared to drastic to have been caused by therapy. The therapist felt uneasy at the sight of this said, "good" little creature. Another parameter was used. The mother's therapist was called and asked to find out what was going on at home, because Carrie's behavior seemed too subdued, even taking into account her newly emerged guilt reactions.

The therapist was upset at this request. She felt she would have to be too directive in her technique and that we were interfering in the life of this family too much. She did find out that Carrie put lotion on the mother's back after the mother's bath in order to relieve a serious psoriasis that was Mrs. A.'s newest symptom. The therapist believed this role-reversal to be detrimental to Carrie.

When she again bathed the doll with such tender yet tense care, she was asked whom she was bathing. "Nobody," she answered. "What's her name?" she was asked again, in the

hope of keeping down the confrontational aspect of the interpretations. Carrie this time shrieked, "Nobody," scooped up
two glasses full of water and poured them on the floor. The attempt to bring this aspect of her relationship with her mother
into the therapeutic setting seemed headed for uncontrollable
regression. Carrie poured more and more water on the floor
and became increasingly agitated. During the next few sessions
Carrie would neither play with the toys nor look at the therapist
but only giggle maniacally at times, rush into the bathroom,
and bring water out to pour on the floor.

Finally she was informed that her therapist did not like the
floor so wet, and that she would have to wipe it up. She just giggled and continued her game. "Not wet," was her answer.

The maniacal giggling and impenetrable agitated behavior
stayed with her for many sessions. The interpretation, "You
would like to make peepee on my floor," brought some relief,
but she kept insisting that the water she poured was not wet.
Strangely enough, there were not complaints from her mother.
Apparently the delusions were reserved for the therapist. While
she was pouring the water, she often made movements with her
hands as though she were smoothing out something or building
up a sandpile.

The agitation subsided somewhat after repeated interpretations of the water as urine. She became willing to play
other games, to continue with the body image songs and exercises, etc., when she began to realize that the therapist could be
neither destroyed nor made angry by the pouring of water.

However, the ritual of pouring water and at times literally
flooding the floor became a great inconvenience. After putting
up with it for about a month (and taking a good look at her own
countertransference) the therapist decided that Carrie would
have to be taught to understand the reality aspect of the situation, that the water was indeed wet, and water, not urine.

Carrie's sense of touch was excellent. It had been used to
explore the surroundings and had achieved good results. She
could easily translate the feeling experiences into words: indeed, during the time when she had touched and felt many ob-

jects, her vocabulary had grown amazingly. The therapist determined that at the next pouring, this method would have to be used. So when she began the ritual again, the therapist picked her up and sat her down on the wet floor, right in the middle of the puddle. A startled look crossed her face. "It's wet," she said. "Yes, it's wet," was the answer. "Can't go to the beach any more," she informed her therapist, and settled down to wiping up the mess, something she had never been willing to do before. It was hoped that at a later date it might be possible to work on the appearance of omnipotent aggression the therapist's action must have conveyed.

Later, her mother said that Carrie's favorite summer past-time had been to go to the beach, but that at one time she had nearly drowned when wading too deep into the water. Her mother had severely punished her after this incident and told her she could not come to the beach any more if she didn't learn to stay out of the deep water.

Had Carrie's flooding of the therapy room been an attempt to drown the therapist, had it been an attempt to master anxiety by recreating the dangerous situation, or was it an attempt to internalize the warning of the mother and to establish some sort of superego? One can only speculate. The symptom occurred once more, when the therapist prepared to take her vacation in the summer. Carrie once again began to flood the floor but said that she could not believe that the therapist would ever return.

Upon the therapist's return from vacation, Carrie became very tractable but was convinced that she was a dirty girl with a smelly "gina." She still bathed dolls, and on occasion drowned them. However, more and more of her bizarre behavior had been brought under control and manifested itself in an inability to take direction, excessive shyness, and occasional temper tantrums.

In the sessions she was now able to "dance." Carrie would hop or bounce, stop, and look at her therapist expectantly until she was imitated. Sometimes the therapist and Carrie would play hopping-bouncing-running together and accompany themselves with rhythmic sounds. "Bopbopbop" was for hopping. "Pppppp" was for bouncing, and a long drawn "aaaahhh" for running. They made up songs and silly games that had them both giggling and laughing and rolling on the floor. Mrs. A. commented that they seemed to be making a lot of noise.

After the long period of getting acquainted and learning to trust, Carrie now wanted to hear music. Until this phase was ushered in, Carrie wanted to do everything alone. But now, she took pleasure in walking fast or slow to appropriate music, doing the "Alley Cat" and playing Ring-around-the-rosy with the therapist.

Her parents took this as a cue that Carrie could enter kindergarten. In the therapist's opinion, she was not ready to do so. She was too fragile to cope with long absences from home just yet. But her mother was basking in Carrie's new ability to kiss and hug, to laugh and talk. She simply couldn't see that Carrie wasn't ready yet. Despite lengthy explanations, she entered Carrie in a special class for developmentally disabled children. The expectable happened. Carrie spent several weeks crying desperately. She clung to her therapist in her sessions and didn't want to leave. Mrs. A. became furious. Carrie had to go to school, the teacher agreed with her, and that was that. Eventually Carrie gave in. She curled up in a fetal position, stuck her thumb in her mouth, and remained that way until the school decided they couldn't handle her. At home, however, she behaved well.

At this point, Mrs. A. dropped her own therapy. She felt it no longer served her. She also had grave doubts about Carrie's treatment. She was told that Carrie could not be expected to do all the changing alone, that she needed reinforcement at home, no punishment. But 4 years of therapy for mother and child had not produced enough for Carrie's parents. She had learned to talk and interact with her family, bizarre gesturing and hallucinatory behavior had disappeared, but she was still fragile and prone to regressions. Her manipulative withdrawal was proof of failure to her parents. Carrie was withdrawn from therapy. Subsequently, her parents sought and received placement for Carrie in a day-treatment center for severely emotionally disturbed children. There Carrie was viewed as high-functioning and suitable for psychotherapy. But her parents were thoroughly alienated by that idea and reverted to the view that Carrie must be neurologically impaired, despite evidence to the contrary.

For this writer, it had to be enough that Carrie had become a thoroughly human if eccentric little girl, who would not ever have to face the threat of hospitalization that hung over her at the beginning of the interaction.

Symbols of the Maternal Breast Used by Three Schizophrenic Teenagers

Tom, Marty, and Marcia came to dance-movement therapy as chronologic teenagers, but their developmental level was far from that. They were stuck, or fixated in the symbiotic stage of development, or were so overstimulated by either external or internal events that tension release, or homeostasis, did not take place. This is believed to have occurred during so early a time in life that ''mother'' as a whole object had not yet emerged from the undifferentiated, boundaryless state of ''symbiosis.'' It became clear very soon that they experienced interpersonal relationships only as supply or lack of food, namely a ''breast'' or part object.

All three teenagers presented an inability to express themselves freely, and complained that they could not defend themselves. All three also wanted to be able to dance rock and roll with their peers without feeling ''embarrassed and uptight.''

In the two boys, reality testing and contact with the objective world had either been partially restored during previous psychotherapy or had never been lost completely, while the girl was frequently subject to hallucinations and visions.

Physically, the three were of adequate development. Medical tests revealed no deficiencies.

Despite a fairly wide age span—the boys being thirteen and nineteen, the girl, seventeen—and of their totally differing skeletal structures, they exhibited similar postures and movement patterns. They also suffered from marked anxiety symptoms, such as uneven breathing patterns, fidgeting, flicking of hands, and heavy perspiring during the beginning and end of each movement therapy session.

Withdrawal and denial were the defense mechanisms most often employed.

The similarity in posture consisted of a slight stoop in the shoulders, a forward bend in the upper part of the spine that in Marcia's case was so pronounced as to be disturbing to her family who referred to it as a "widow's hump." (As an aside, this term showed quite a bit of unconscious insight into Marcia's pathology).

This depressive slump of the shoulders and spine narrowed the rib cage of all three and forced shallow, inadequate breathing patterns. Although by no means obese, the three had "tires" around their middles, protruding abdomens, and shuffling walks. Both posture and walk improved during treatment, not only because growing self-esteem allowed a straightening of the spine but also because resolution of the breast fixations made the taking in air as a food equivalent pleasurable.

Both boys liked to stand with their legs crossed over each other, protecting their genitals, in a truly precarious balance, as though the price they had to pay for protecting themselves was their equilibrium. They often joked about these things, but did not give them up until they had become aware of the underlying equations and fixations.

Marcia often spent minutes looking at her therapist's breasts, then touched her own chest area, only to shake her head mournfully as if to indicate either that she was not aware that she had breasts or that they were defective in some way. She began verbalizing these fears at the time she became acquainted with her ambivalence toward the introjected maternal breast.

Another similarity was an almost total inability to hear a

beat and to translate it into a simple bounce or even to tap it with foot or hand. Apparently the taking in and using of rhythms was perceived as dangerous, in the same way that the intake of air had to be shallow in order to avoid anxiety. The equation Mother's Milk-Air-Rhythmic Sound emerged clearly during breathing and relaxing exercises.

Tom

Tom, thirteen, reacted to the whole idea of movement therapy with great hostility. Having to look at and imitate the therapist immediately aroused a set of fears which he verbalized with great facility, so great a facility, indeed, that their defensive aspects were in the forefront. Endowed with an exceptionally high I.Q. and an amazing ability to remember details, he used these functions for hiding maneuvers, especially against the possible intrusion of a lady ''who doesn't know as much as a psychiatrist.'' While talking about how smart some people are or are not and how he wished he were already in college where people would be more adult and not attack him physcially or make him feel bad about his inability to punch or defend himself effectively with his fists, he finally abreacted enough anxiety to let go temporarily of his crosslegged, unsteady posture to look directly at the therapist. She was moving in a simplified waltz pattern to music from *Sleeping Beauty*. This music was chosen for its smooth, waving quality and strong repetitious beat, since Tom had become almost paralyzed with fear when his own choice, *Love me, love me, do* by the Beatles, had been played in a previous session.

His muscles became literally like rocks when confronted by the fulfillment of his wish to dance to that particular song.

It is easy enough to state that wish-fulfillment early in a therapeutic relationship it too anxiety-provoking and that willingness to ''love'' him by granting his request, as the title of the record suggested, was too much of a treat in his hazy constellation of shaky object relationships; or even that he sexualized any attempt to dance with him in a manner suggested by him.

It may have been a combination of all these factors that drove him to so drastic a response.

He stood in his typical position, rigid, unable to move, staring at the therapist with unseeing eyes as though he could make himself disappear by immobility. Eventually, he began to sway backward, almost imperceptibly, as though the rigor of controlling himself and his feelings so tightly had finally taken on a life of its own and was moving him out of the presumably malevolent sphere of the therapist's influence. A steadying hand was offered. He evaded it quickly and blurted out: "I'm a weakling. I can't do anything right." At the same time he clenched and unclenched his fists.

The ambience of expected terror, projected onto the therapist from long ago, was still so strong that she decided to ask Tom simply to walk in a circle. This was done primarily to give him a chance to relax the still visible rigidity in his previously tightened muscles by performing a simple, non-threatening task, and secondly to convey that his anxiety and hostility were accepted and were not seen as frightening. The therapist would not force him to give up either until he was willing to do so. Apparently he understood the nonverbal interpretation immediately.

"You don't want me to punch, or anything?" he asked. "Why do you want me to walk? I know how to walk. I'm no baby."

Still complaining loudly, he began to walk in a circle, after a while recovering the natural coordination of arms and legs swinging in opposition. Slowly even his stiff feet relaxed and for a short moment one could see a naturally flowing walk, with feet arching strongly and flexibly.

Tom's playing dead, making himself immobile when given what he asked for, alerted the therapist to the deep resentment and fear of a feeding situation this boy must be covering up. His verbalization appeared to indicate some awareness of anger and a need to cope with it—"Don't you want me to punch"—as well as a denial of a strong dependency need—"I'm no baby."

Muscular relaxation would have to be brought about

gradually, to avoid panic reactions and to allow for sufficient reintegration of energy, once, step by step, those strata in his life were reached where the habitual withdrawals and rigidities had been formed.

Tom's reaction to the waltz pattern was less dramatic but equally informative. He managed to produce a fair equivalent, and for a short time dreamily allowed himself to sway with the therapist in time to the music. He picked up the timing from her moving less with the record than with little conscious distortions planted in her pattern to test him. Permitting this identification with her movements to occur appeared to be a sign of trust, an acknowledgement that the previous session had not objectively held any terror and that at some time in the future healthy object relations would come to pass. After all, the baby learns about bodies and moving in its mother's arms and later by observing, imitating, taking in, until many details become an incorporated whole.

The work continued in this pattern for some time. Any attempt made to gratify any of Tom's nonverbal or verbalized needs was met with rigidity and alarm, while little by little his ability to copy simple body image exercises, such as angel-in-the-snow and the *port des bras* of the ballet class, increased, provided the music had an easy, steady flow and the therapist's movements stayed even and large.

A large bouncer ball was also employed. Tom would perch timidly on it hanging on to the handles with all his might, and lurch across the room sitting on it, as though he were afraid of breaking something.

The quality of his behavior was not mentioned to him but he was shown how to use his thigh muscle more effectively and how to make the natural bounce of the ball propel him forward. The bouncer eventually provided the vehicle, both figuratively and concretely, for the next step in development.

While trying to jump higher on the bouncer, Tom bumped into the therapist throwing her off balance.

"Did I hurt you? Did I hurt you? Did you break something?" he wailed.

The therapist demonstrated that she was hale and hearty but added, verbally, that she thought him quite strong.

"Strong? Only because the monster helped me. I'm not strong."

This was the first time he had ever given the bouncer a name. Then he stroked it, caressed it, leaned on it, tried to balance on it, with a little sideways glance at his therapist licked it, and in general comported himself as though the "monster" were the source of his strength.

Finally, with a joyous shout, he decided to play cowboy and rider, waving an imaginary lasso in the air and performing a complete rodeo of wrestling and riding the "monster."

When the hour came to an end, he asked: "Did you fake it or did you really have to fall?"

He was assured that the therapist had indeed responded to the impact of his bump. Suddenly his exhilaration vanished. He sat down on the floor to tie his sneakers, flicked his hands, grimaced, tried not to end the session.

"You don't want to leave," his therapist offered.

"I'm not strong out there," he mumbled, and ran out as fast as he could after revealing so much.

His initial play with the bouncer after throwing his therapist off balance had much the same quality as an infant romping with his mother on the floor. It had the same spontaneous, experimental air. But was mother really "a monster" in his universe? The way he had fondled and licked and kicked and kneaded the ball had been an illustration of how he felt about the breast that had not supplied all his needs, that was indeed a source of strength and of food but was also a "monster" that withheld and threatened.

The tacit approval of his performance had spurred him on to more grown-up things: he gave vent to his exhibitionistic, phallic needs and became a "big boy" who could show off and be strong for an approving mother figure. A "big boy," certainly, but still one who believed in magic, who was strong only in the studio.

From then on the bouncer became an important part of

each session. Tom discovered that the heavy rubber was both soft and strong and speculated, full of wonder, how that could be. He experimentally squeezed the therapist's arm, felt his own biceps, and finally decided that both were soft and strong.

His ability to hear and use rhythms improved now, and the anxious behavior at the beginning of each session vanished. Separation anxiety at the end was still pronounced. Small wonder, for who would want to leave a place of magic strength.

He began to do tribal dancing with the therapist. He was instructed to use the sacrum correctly, to lean the torso slightly forward, to bend knees and to bounce them up and down to strong drum beats and African chants.

Tom revelled in making up hunting dances, war dances, all based on a wide open second position bounce. He imitated karate experts, spear throwers, and warriors but would not execute any of his choreography along. The therapist had to accompany him on all his imaginary exploits and show him the "correct way." Even when she just danced along with him, he would devour each movement with his eyes and adjust his movement as closely as possible to hers.

His positive transference was evident, although the therapist was not allowed to initiate any new dances or fantasy games. He needed her to be his mirror, the reinforcer of his newfound strength.

The bouncer was treated more impersonally now. It served as horse or chariot, or sometimes as a missile. Tom mastered his fear of the loud, smacking noise the big ball made but was concerned that it might break the floor, the walls, or even the therapist. When the record player skipped, Tom thought this was the result of his having thrown the bouncer at it. He was afraid of punishment and destruction of his own body. He began to pound the walls with his fists to test them and asked the therapist to tell his parents that he needed a punching bag in order "to toughen himself up." He began to turn the lights on and off many times, explaining that "he was controlling it."

Finally, he could bear the anxiety no longer. His whole imaginary universe, based in the studio, appeared threatened by destruction.

Tom's aggressive and hostile impulses became centered on the bouncer from which he eventually turned all his world destruction fantasies back onto himself in order to save those nearest and dearest to himself from death and mutilation.

When all this overwhelming emotion reached its wavelike crest, Tom needed to act it out. He had to do something and follow his strong motor drive. Placing a battered plastic bat on the floor, he rode the bouncer on top of it and smashed it to smithereens with his riding.

"I killed it," he announced.

"You think you killed it," the therapist responded.

"What's death?" he wanted to know. "If I hold my breath long enough, I'll faint. Maybe I'll die. Or maybe I'll have brain damage from holding my breath. My mother thinks I have brain damage, that's why I act so nutty."

He wanted to give a demonstration of breath-holding which he claimed was a competitive game among "some guys he knew."

Instead, deep breathing exercises were suggested, the exact opposite of what he supposedly wanted. The results were startling. In between taking deep breaths and climbing on the desk to open the window above it, Tom explained that one's vision blurs when holding one's breath, that one could black out, even while in bed, that falling into a deep pit was really the same as not breathing.

He revealed the whole range of oral incorporative fears. Had the hat he killed been symbolic of his mother's withholding breasts?

On a reality level, Tom's mother had defended herself against a diagnosis of schizophrenia for Tom by stating that he must have brain damage, that he was odd even as a baby.

Finally, Tom had revealed enough. He settled into deep, controlled breathing, hungrily drinking in as much air as possible. On leaving, he remarked: "My brain shouldn't be enemies with my body."

After the session in which he had "killed it," there was no more mention of any fear that walls and floor might break, or any indication that he thought of himself and his activities as dangerous. Apparently these fears had served as a defense against an even deeper, more primitive one, which, however, had not yet come fully to the surface.

He would also often break into small, spontaneous war dances that always involved some smooth plastic pillows.

After one of his improvisations, during which he displayed total body movement, he began to kick and punch the largest of them. He seemed to forget that he was not alone in the room. He repeated this performance several times, until it became clear that there was more than muscular tension, possibly built by the fatiging jumps and leaps of his war dance, being abreacted.

He turned unseeing eyes to the therapist and mumbled: "You expect it to burst. But it doesn't. It just throws you off."

He began to tremble. His face crumpled and for a moment seemed ready to cry. Instead, he asked for a drink of water. He was given some. While he drank it, Brahm's *Lullabye* was played to calm him. He drank the water, then leaned against the therapist, put his arms around her and rocked her, showing her what kind of mother he had wanted when he was a hungry, desperate infant.

Tom was scheduled to go to camp soon. He used the remaining month well. He kicked and punched the pillow, but in a directed way. Eventually, the pillow gave up its ghost, burst at the seams and was not mourned by Tom. He turned his attention to the therapist instead. With a sly, sideways grin he informed her: "You could double for the Pillsbury Doughboy, the way your chest is built."

"Boys don't have chest like mine," she countered.

"Naah. You're a lady," he answered, and turned beet-red. Tom clearly had begun to see his therapist as a whole person, one with a chest. Tom relived the terrible baby rages in which the breast, as part object, was the recipient of all his oral sadistic impulses. Once he had gotten the after-effects of this rage out of his body and been able to discard the muscular defenses against the re-emergence of his terrible aggression, he was able to straighten up and to relate to his therapist, and to the world, in a more complete and free way.

Marty

Marty presented himself for his first session with a considerable amount of surface poise. A chunky young man of nineteen with huge biceps and unusually large thigh muscles, he emphasized the shortness of his neck by raising and pushing his shoulders slightly forward. As an opener, he had brought a notebook full of poems for which he had received praise from both his former psychotherapist and his English teacher.

When he handed the notebook over, he stood in the same stance Tom used to take, only instead of a loose-jointed will-o-the-wisp, he appeared to have the ease and solidity of an athelete. His left leg was turned out at the hip and planted with equally turned out foot on the floor. The right leg was crossed over, protecting his genitals, the weight of the leg resting on the toe. However, the weight shifting that should have taken place to make such a posture secure had not occurred.

Seeing the general direction of my glance, he quickly placed himself on both legs and said: "My pants are tight. Next time, I'll wear looser ones." The comment seemed to express an awareness that the posture served defensive purposes.

Work was started with a few simple gymnastic and body image exercises. The results were disheartening. Muscular Marty, an accomplished track runner, with a long history of working out in the gym, could only raise his arms above his head with the greatest difficulty, and experienced anxiety attacks while asked to kick or to open his arms. He appeared incapable of reproducing simple dance steps, though he did hear and was able to tap out rhythms on the floor. However, all his movements had a jerky, forced quality as though the strength of his muscles were not viable but got in his way. He was able to walk on his toes and could hold *releve* for many beats, an ability that became less pronounced as his muscles lost some of their rigidity. The "stoniness," the momentary petrification observed in Tom, was habitual in Marty, although not carried to the same degree as in Tom.

At the end of the first session, Marty made a long list of requests. He didn't want to do any "ballet stuff" but asked for a whole lesson built around *grands battements*. The therapist's had looked like knives to him, he said, and he wanted that for himself. He knew he stood and walked incorrectly. Could he be shown how to look taller and how to dance rock and roll. While he spoke his face became puffy and red, his body even more rigid, fully expecting the therapist to deny each and every one of his urgent requests as angrily as he made them.

He was assured that the therapist had heard everything he said. Discussing details might have added fuel to his aggressive greed.

In order to make new movement patterns available to Marty, relaxing and breathing exercises would be essential, since the rigidity in his muscles appeared to be a habitual warding off of new and possibly distrubing experiences. Part of each session was spent in Autogenic Training and with the, simple breathing exercises swimmers use.

The conscious relaxing of body parts had a good effect on Marty. Instead of getting sleepy, he would suddenly get up and announce: "Let's work now," or "I'm ready to dance."

He never let a session go by without asking for "that kicking music," meaning the appropriate band for *grand battements* on a ballet teacher's record. Somehow he never managed to lock his knees or hold his upper body straight and complained bitterly about not being able to achieve the proper knifelike effect. This, incidentally, was the only exercise during which he ever looked at the therapist directly. Sometimes, he would watch her in the mirror and pick up a pattern that way. When asked to repeat something, or to perform himself, he would either turn his back or clutch at the barre for support at the expense of distorting combinations designed for the center.

Nevertheless, he was able to take in a great deal of what was offered. The therapist theorized that at that time she represented the feeding, but penetrating and potentially dangerous breast. That he was unable to take in or imitate the aggressive,"knifelike" *grand battements* seemed further proof that for the time being any recognition of the full range of human emotions, and complete interpersonal relationships were out of the question. Arabesques, or simply stepping toward the therapist were also anxiety-provoking, as though coming any closer would mean either being devoured or having to devour me himself. The term "devour" seems particularly appropriate here since during such exercises Marty would open his mouth slightly and begin to salivate until tremors and heavy perspiring would signal that the anxiety level was becoming uncontrollable. He would then visibly "pull himself together" by tightening his muscles.

A little comment from the therapist such as "It's okay," or a pat on his shoulder appeared to help him. More sympathy than just these meager tokens frightened him.

After several months of diligent work, Marty came in extremely depressed. He had lost his best friend. Why? When they went out to drink beer and "to pick up chicks" Marty had used a "bad" word and that had "turned his friend off." Looking utterly crestfallen, he insisted that now he was all alone. He would enlarge neither on what had happened between him and his friend nor did he seem able to remember the existence of his large and devoted family.

After pacing the studio distractedly, his face puffy and distorted, Marty came up with an idea. Could he have the kicking music and could he dance out to it, what he really felt about his friend?

Standing in second position, one hand on the barre, bent slightly forward and tight as a metal coil, Marty was ready for attack. The music played loudly, inviting aggression. Marty stood motionless, a slight flush moving up his neck. The music reached a crescendo. No action from Marty. A convulsive tremor of the type described by Alexander Lower (1967), travelled up his calves. Then, as the music reached its last, familiar tremolo, Marty stretched out his arm, pointed his finger half-heartedly into a corner, saying accusingly, "Shame, shame."

Tears streaming down his face, he sobbed: "I can't. Anyway, I don't care. Who needs him anyway." His shoulders were pulled up even higher than usual, his neck a solid fold under a glistening, puffy face. He looked like a turtle about to disappear forever inside its shell. The time for intervention had come.

"This is a safe place, Marty," the therapist told him, and put the music back on. Marty got the message. With strong, decisive thrusts, he began pounding the wall with his fists again and again, as though trying systematically to pound a universe into shape. He stopped when the music did. "Again," he said, "Kicking now," This time there was no trouble with *grands battements*. Up they came, out they shot, properly placed and rhythmically spaced.

"Will you be here?" he asked when he left, his shoulders relaxed and his spine straight.

During the next session Marty acted like a turtle *without* a shell. He came in, spine straight and shoulders relaxed, but head down, and he wanted to hold the therapist's hand, as though in supplication.

"You didn't hurt me," she responded. "I wasn't angry at you," his reply came quickly, out of his throat, with no breath behind it. She repeated, "I'm fine. You didn't hurt me." Whereupon he spilled it all out.

He had wished on his friend that the Viet Cong would get him when the friend called him a draft-dodger. He didn't have the right to wish death on anyone. And then, did the therapist guess his dream every night? There it was again, that belief in magic powers and, by inference, the magic of his own aggression which might kill by wishing alone.

The information that the therapist knew nothing of the contents, or even the fact of his dreaming, amazed Marty. He walked around her thoughtfully. "You can't read it in my muscles?" Another thoughtful inspection trip around her.

"Why not?" "I'm no magician."

"But you know when I'm angry, and when I feel bad. You know when to make me cry and when to make me breathe."

In answer, he was led to the mirror. The therapist demonstrated some of his typical positions. "I know, because it feels the same way to me," she said. Laughingly he joined her "Head up" he told himself. "I look taller that way."

From his therapist making him do things, controlling him as the infant feels controlled by his own impulses as well as by his mother, Marty had grown to accept responsibility for his own posture.

From then on, Marty provided his own music. He favored B. B. King's soulful wailing about betrayed males and faithless females, remarking that B. B. King "knew the same way the therapist knew." "Knowing" in Marty's sense had something to do with magically sensing someone else's feelings.

The sessions began to look much like a modern jazz class as we strutted and trucked and hunched our shoulder and gyrated our pelvic areas. Marty had little trouble picking up combinations and even began to improvise a little. The only area that really remained "uptight" was his hip and pelvis. He claimed that the girls he picked up in dance halls and bars liked his dancing but rebuffed his sexual advances. He glanced at the therapist adoringly and a bit in awe during such times. Eventually he began to bring in small gifts and wrote poems especially for her.

"You are looking for a girlfriend who is like me." She interpreted as she again refused to accept an offering. He looked more like a small, embarrassed schoolboy when he brought presents than like a young man practicing to be a suitor in the real world.

He accepted the verbal interpretation with the same docility with which he offered gifts and danced. He also found dancing in the center too frightening and asked for a longer time at the barre. All this time he worked diligently. A lengthening and softening of the hard bunches of muscles in his arms and legs, as well as a deepening of his breathing pattern occurred.

Eventually, however, the constant wailing of blues in the session began to create an atmosphere that was no longer conducive to growth. Marty seemed to have settled all too comfortably into an imagined world of faithlessness and impotence.

There was something in the way Mary responded physically to the music after a while that seemed astereotyped and too comfortable, as though he were substituting someone else's sighs for his own.

The next time he came, *Swan Lake* was put on the record player. Marty listened, then bowed to the therapist in the classic manner. Was he going to dance the prince to her Swan Queen? He picked up the thought immediately and began to posture and prance in imitation of that classic and much abused ballet.

Finally, he held out his hand. Gravely, the therapist responded and together, in perfect time, they danced *chasse, chasse, assemble, assemble,* and then broke into a waltz. For that short time, they merged into a remarkable unit that responded perfectly to the music and each other.

It was hard for Marty to go home after that. The therapist wondered how he would be able to integrate such an experience of closeness to another human being. She didn't have to wait long for an answer. He telephoned that same day to cancel his next session. He was dizzy and nauseated, and ready to quit. The merging had, for him, been devouring of the therapist, hence the nausea.

He was told squarely that one didn't quit over the phone, that one had to face one's therapist to do that. He agreed to come and slunk in the next time puffy-faced and ready to be killed for what he considered to be an offense. After all, hadn't he symbolically killed the therapist twice, once in the dance by merging with her and once by trying to get rid of her over the phone?

He sat on the floor and seemed ready to cry. After a long silence he confided the following dream. He was spinning in empty space, around and around until he finally was shattered by a large round moutain. "Like this?" the therapist asked and began to spin like a dervish turning on her own axis. Grudgingly, Marty consented to try: nothing. He couldn't even turn once. But his interest was engaged again. He agreed not to leave until he could spin.

It took Marty a good month of steady work, but he learned

how to spin, up and down his own axis, regaining footing and momentum time and again. Eventually he fell to the floor exhausted, but instead of sprawling wide open, he curled up in a fetal position and began to whimper, "I'm thirsty." The therapist brought him water which he drank greedily. Then he simply put his head in her lap and stayed there till the end of the hour.

He had finally reached the fixation point and found that no mountain breast waited to disintegrate his being, but that the environment, far from being hostile, would support, nourish, and cherish him.

Marcia

Marcia's pathology was a good deal more obvious than the boys. She had not been able to maintain herself in public school. The parents had resisted suggestion that she be placed in a residential institution, so the girl's formal education had come to an end when she was in the eighth grade. She had been under the care of a psychoanalytically oriented psychiatrist, who felt that movement therapy might help her to overcome, or at least to halt, an increasingly bizarre gait and posture and that it might promote the development of a more adequate body image. He felt he could no longer help her. Marcia seemed unaware of, or at the very least enormously ambivalent toward her own ample breasts.

Marcia's family, too, had trouble accepting the diagnosis of schizophrenia and preferred to justify her odd and sometimes asocial behavior as mental retardation. However, at the onset of her psychosis, the school psychologist had obtained an I.Q. score of 97; this was after she had already been unable to do her work properly in the fifth grade.

The parents had joined a local association for retarded children and under the auspices of that organization, Marcia regularly attended bimonthly teen dances. There she became much interested in dancing the new rock and roll creations and indeed taught herself to sling her awkward bulk about in creditable imitations of all the latest fads. She also became interested in the Beatles, who were her idols, learned all their songs by heart, and spent hours at home listening to their records.

She did not endear herself to the other youngsters at the dances since she caustically and very often correctly commented on their inabilities. She felt they were ugly, mean, and "after" her, thus displacing the anger she felt toward her mother onto her hapless companions.

The thought of having in the therapist a constant dance partner pleased Marcia. At the first meeting, she hugged her, asked if she could call her by her first name, and, in general, comported herself like a toddler at Christmas who is delighted by all the gifts but simultaneously frightened by the thought that they might all disappear.

While dancing to her favorite record *Shake it up, baby* it was noted that she used her legs as though she had no knees and that there was a similar petrification in her wrists which she relieved on occasion by flicking her hands. At times of tension, her fingers were crossed and intertwined until they resembled nothing so much as a triangle of popsicle sticks. Every once in a while she would rhythmically, and in time with the music, stab this triangle into the general direction of her breasts and then her vaginal area, without, however, ever really coming close to either.

Her walk was a peculiar limping shuffle which favored the right side and reinforced the picture of an old widow already clearly shown by her "widow's hump."

Since both her equilibrium and her walk were so poorly coordinated, work was begun sitting on the floor. In this position, on the floor, Marcia learned about spatial relationships such as up, down, back and front in relationship to her own body, as well as the balletic *port de bras*.

In order to make use of Marcia's enthusiasm for music, the therapist soon began to employ Strauss Waltzes. Unable to move even a single step without getting hopelessly tangled up, Marcia moved simply and sweetly and correctly when allowed to put her arms around the therapist's neck and to place her head against her shoulder. Like a very young child, she picked rhythm and pattern up by body contact. For a long time there was no carry-over once she let go, though there was always a general softening of her tensions right after the waltzes, and for a short time she could perform more adequately. During these few minutes she resembled a satiated infant, who, one with its world after being rocked and fed by mother, is willing to do anything for her.

Many fruitful sessions followed during which Marcia learned to accept her body as her own. However, running and jumping exercises scared her.

Eventually, she supplied the reason. After a particularly successful set of jumps, she pointed to her breasts and said: "That's too personal. They wiggle-waggle. Mustn't touch. That's not what my mother is paying for."

"All women have breasts," she was reassured.

"Mustn't touch," she repeated shamefacedly, and performed her particular set of pointing and flicking.

"You think you should not touch your vagina," the therapist ventured.

"That's not what my mother is paying for," said Marcia, and for the first time rushed from the room.

The therapist assumed that she meant mother's introjected prohibition was being lifted. Apparently she had understood a warning against masturbation as a warning against growing up as well. The link between becoming aware of her breasts as part of herself and the simultaneous pointing toward her vaginal area symbolized this.

During her next session, Marcia didn't want to do her clinch around the therapist's neck and waltz. She seemed determined to clarify something.

"You said bad words," she informed the therapist, flicked and pointed, and then stared fixedly out of the window.

"Breast and vagina are the names of those body parts," was the answer.

"The leaves are stirring," mentioned Marcia defensively,

and started to sway and waltz like one herself. Her very first improvisation was enjoyable but recognizable as defensive. In order not to have to talk more, Marcia danced alone, using her extremeties gracefully and in an organized way.

Finally, she attempted a backbend and came up giggling and embarrassed because her breasts had "wiggle-waggled" again.

"My grandmother gave them to me," she declared and cupped her breasts with her hands.

The therapist formulated that Marcia danced by herself, as a separate entity, who still had to please a threatening maternal figure by showing what she had learned and who could acknowledge stirred feelings only in metaphors: "The leaves are stirring."

One day, quite casually, Marcia informed the therapist the reason her breasts were so ample was that she was pregnant. She further insisted that she had to be fat and pregnant now, because when she had been slimmer she was always dizzy.

"Dizzy like falling," she said. "That's why I used to walk crazy, I could fall from being dizzy."

She was talking to me about the same oral incorporative fears that Marty and Tom had so vividly re-experienced. Abreaction was unnecessary because repression had barely taken place. She had lived out the fear of falling from the breast daily and in order to defend herself against annihiliation, had denied the existence of her own breasts and had adjusted her walk to keep upright. Now, during a time in treatment roughly corresponding to the separation-individuation phase, as described by Mahler, she was able to verbalize her experiences. She also had to deny that her mother had given birth to her. "My grandmother gave them (the breasts) to me," was an expression of the fear and rejection she felt for her mother, whom she perceived as not wanting her to grow up.

During later months it was discovered during some bending exercises that made Marcia aware of her spine that the "widow's hump" was an incorporation of a characteristic of her deceased grandmother. Grandmother had become the parent surrogate who allowed limited growth. It was discussed how good her grandmother had been to her and how she had baked cookies, etc., for Marcia. She now began to ask for cookies and milk from the therapist also. Becoming Marcia's grandmother had its drawbacks. She didn't want to dance any longer but tried to convince the therapist to take on the whole role of grandmother.

After this episode was worked through Marcia's preoccupation with her breasts ceased.

She left therapy when the family moved out of town because the father had accepted a job elsewhere.

In all three cases, skeletomuscular inhibitions were an attempt to express, or to point to, fixation points through constant tension and to control overwhelming aggressive impulses on a physical level.

This symbol of the withholding maternal breast recurred strongly in the treatments of all three clients. Tom employed a battered plastic hat and cushions to show what he felt, Marty dreamed of a round mountain, and Marcia had difficulties with her own breasts. Although many of their ego functions were at a much higher level then, for instance, Carrie's, at the beginning of treatment they could not respond fully to their surroundings until they were able to give up the fantasy of a hostile and unresponsive breast. Because this fantasy had been formed at a nonverbal time in their lives, it was appropriately worked through on a largely nonverbal, body level.

Trying to Heal the Split; Working with Borderline Clients

Many people who are neither clearly neurotic not clearly psychotic present themselves for treatment both privately and in hospital settings. They are usually called "Borderline." But confusion exists about what this term means.

In the literature, and in case histories at clinics and hospitals, such terms appear as "borderline states," (Knight, 1953), "Preschizophrenic peronality structure," (Rapaport, Gill, & Schaefer, 1945), "Psychotic character," (Frosch 1964), "ambulatory schizophrenia," (Hoch & Polatin, 1949), " 'as-if' personality," (Deutsch, 1942), all attempted to describe a group of clients who seemed to present similar syndromes without fitting into recognizable nosologic categories.

To add to the confusion, dance-movement therapists responsible for the treatment of such clients could add only equally confusing data. On occasion, these people's movement patterns appeared to disintegrate significantly, while their usual mode of locomotion, stance, posture, rhythm, tension, flow, effort, (Laban, 1947), and interpersonal dynamic seemed well-integrated.

Furthermore, these disintegrations were not then clearly identifiable as to developmental level, and were not always traceable to experiential stress. Thus, a description of "temporary psychotic break" did not seem out of line, but provided little in the way of a hint toward treatment approach, particularly since recovery was also always abrupt and tenuous, and did not follow a predictable curve.

Since little agreement existed as to origins and etiology of this puzzling behavior pattern, even relatively sophisticated clinicians of many different theoretical backgrounds were tempted into overly enthusiastic prognosis.

Recently, however, some stabilization and theoretical agreement has been reached based on the research by Otto Kernberg which was initially supported by the Menninger Foundation (1966) and was later funded by a Public Health Service Research Grant from the National Institute of Mental Health.

Kernberg's findings are of particular interest here because this group of clients appears to be the second largest referral group in dance-movement therapy. Their frequent loss of body boundaries and strong need for tension discharge fairly cries out for movement intervention.

First and foremost is the important fact that the behavioral vacillations mentioned earlier are part and parcel of a chronic and stable characterologic system having nothing to do with the transitory, acute manifestations of an overt psychotic break.

Thus, the rapid changes in their actions and moods do not appear strange to these clients. Either the changes are not acknowledged at all, or are rationalized as "spontaneity." Since this "spontaneity" is rarely sublimated into joyous and creative living but stays within channels of infantile tension discharge, it is somewhat easier to identify than the other components of the psychic picture under discussion here.

Typically, these clients fail to recognize their difficulties as symptoms, and thus do not appear for treatment until stress forces disintegration, then, during intake interviews, the therapist finds thought processes to be intact again. Primary-process functioning is not apparent until the first nonstructured session with a psychotherapist or during projective tests. Here, in the permissive presence of a possibly significant person, the enormous amount of diffuse, freefloating anxiety always present reveals itself, and many of the phobias related to the body that are always present with Borderline Personality Organization come to the surface. Fear of blushing, of speaking in public, of being looked at, of being contaminated, as well as severe social inhibitions, usually in various combinations, *never* any one phobia by itself, are presumptive evidence for diagnosis of borderline personality functioning. Because of the presence of such multiple resomatization (Schur, 1955), dance-movement therapy is often the treatment of choice.

Kernberg (1975) himself advocates "modified psychoanalytic psychotherapy" as most effective in private practice, including the setting of limits and structuring of sessions, as well as the preservation of the therapist's neutrality. In a hospital setting, less structure is advised, since too strict structure may foster dependency and apathy and/or cover the pathology (Kernberg, 1976). Giovaccini (1972) speaks of a "modified psychoanalytic approach," while Kohut (1971) is in favor of maintaining the classic analytic approach. However, much of Kohut's work refers to a special subgroup of Borderline Organization known as "Narcissistic Personality Disorder," whose difficulties are based on developmental arrests of self-esteem and lack of separation from significant others. (Stolorow

& Lachman, 1980). Kernberg, whos hypothesis is adopted here, speaks more about clinets whose anger at the frustrating parent propelled them into premature internal separation, leaving them both vulnerable and isolated. Never having experienced sufficient amounts of gratification, their need to be loved and admired is enormous. Thus their pathology is more object relational than conflictual.

Also present in Borderline Organization are well-rationalized obsessive rituals and much hypochondriasis with bizarre conversion syptoms which often involve bodily hallucinations and complex sensations.

For instance, one client claimed to meditate extensively, and to reach deep states of relaxation from which she emerged refreshed and happy. Nevertheless, she showed up for her session immediately following her meditations physically tense and cramped in every available skeletal muscle. Relaxation exercises and deep breathing in conjunction with the therapist as well as stretching on the floor and at the barre, eventually enabled the client to differentiate her own bodily sensations sufficiently to admit that she had no control over her "meditations," but experienced a form of twilight state which ennervated her. After many ups and downs in the treatment situation, it eventually become apparent that the "meditations" served to bind an overwhelming rage which had been visible in the muscle tension states all along (Fenichel, 1945). Denial and splitting as defenses were used so forcefully that contradictory feelings were able to exist side by side without being questioned by the clients. This is in line with Kernberg's investigation showing that denial simply reinforces splitting. These clients are aware that they have vacillating views about other people and themselves, but this fact has no emotional meaning for them.

Kernberg also shows that "splitting" as a defense is related to early development, when perception and cognition have not yet reached a level that would permit the intergration of the person or thing as *both* good and bad. Memory traces of both gratification and frustration are stored in normal growth and help to sort out the origin of stimuli as well as their characteristics. Thus, mother and other important persons are recognized as the sources of many different action-reaction cycles. The maturing ego integrates the fact that both positive and negative sensations and feelings can emanate from one and the same source.

In the type of pathology discussed here, however, the mother who said "no" is shoved into a different drawer of the memory compartment than the mother who said, "yes." Thus, one person is seen as actually being two people, each of whom is contacted with a full set of emotional, ideational, and motor consciousness of a contradictory nature.

As long as the contradictions are kept separated and are activated alternately, anxiety is kept at bay. Thus the madly adored person of today can become the completely abhorred person of tomorrow.

During sessions, the transferences obviously also swing rapidly from total idealization of the therapist to declarations that she does no good at all. She is accused of wasting time with her single-minded devotion to movement that the clients in their own opinion can already execute perfectly with full range of detail. Like all transferences, these swings are a mirror of the client's past and present mode of interpersonal relationships. Here there is no real sense of love or concern for the loved object. The idealized and supposedly loved person is treated ruthlessly as an extension of the client. If the loved one does not allow control and exploitation, he or she is simply discarded or viewed as a hated individual with the need for the alternate side of the coin arises again.

When these contradictory feeling storms arise, the therapist is well advised to keep sessions on an even keel. It needs to be pointed out that since the client felt differently yesterday, there might be a change again tomorrow. Improvisation is best avoided during such times, since unstructured flow of movement frees instinctual material which the oscillating client cannot integrate adequately just then. Empathetic mirroring and strong rhythmic activity aided by whatever music the client has shown a liking for usually brings about a strengthening of body boundaries for the time being. Both the predictable time span and countable beats of recorded music establish a sense of time while mirroring reinforces self-esteem.

It has been observed that the most outstanding movement characteristic during contradictory swings is a speed-up of existing patterns until they become distorted. The whole human movement repertoire appears to be available, but is discarded and disjointed in rapid succession. Clients cannot allow the sessions to flow organically, but claim they do not wish it to progress. They try, and throw out everything and nothing completely and finally announce they don't want dance-movement-therapy anyway. Patient investigation then usually elicits the client's unintegrated, unstable feeling of self. As they alternately over- and undervalue all significant people in their lives, so they over- and undervalue themselves. They might feel dreadfully embarrassed about being looked at, yet blush constantly, and thus pull attention to themselves. They might talk of how insecure and unworthy they feel, but at the same time claim special dispensations from expected behavior because they are also worthier than others.

The opposing statements about the self reflect the fact that neither omnipotent, grandiose fantasies, nor realistic successes have influenced the helplessness and perceived weakness of earlier developmental levels. The basic body image is not experienced as a whole entity, but swings from a libidinal, self-accepting core, to a nucleus of self-destructive, defeatist, not to say autoaggressive feelings which surface as hypochandriasis, body phobias, and lack of trust in interpersonal relationships. The swings from one to the other extreme seem to be triggered by misunderstood bodily responses to events and moods. Close observation as to recognizable quality of response can eventually be shared with the clients so they will learn to view themselves realistically, and weigh their somatic reactions against what actually occurs. Since the ability to test reality is always unimpaired, the client is usually willing to undertake this arduous task *after* the first few swings in the transference have been weathered and trust has been established.

There is some evidence that a constitutionally determined lack of frustration tolerance is present with a subsequent overdevelopment of the aggressive drive (Kernberg, 1976). Therefore the above mentioned measures have to be instituted to acquaint the client with the consequences of his or her behavior. Because of the predominance of splitting, however, such educative means remain unproductive unless self image and interpersonal relationships can be integrated therapeutically at the same time. Obviously, structure and reality orientation are not an intrusive, martial law enforced upon the client. These measures are used to safeguard impulse-ridden clients from destructive behavior, when they are not yet ready to hear interpretations.

Lisi, for instance, presented herself at work seductively yet innocently in low-cut dresses and leotards. She could not understand why men responded with lust to her voluptuous figure. Extremely friendly, she spoke to anyone at all on the street and was incensed when anyone tried to seduce her. During the second year of treatment her improvisations became more and more revealing. She danced as though she were a harem girl who wishes to catch her sultan's eye. Unfortunately, it was only the therapist who witnessed her sensuous invitations. Lisi stormed.

"What good are you? You are not a man."

She began to phone between sessions to talk about men who had found her attractive, and related that she invited some of them up to her apartment. She was then reliving her original disappointment with her mother who had forbidden access to her father by jealous scenes whenever little Lisi tried to get close to him. Lisi could not acknowledge the painful happenings from her past until she was firmly told that her present actions could lead to rape. Lisi's eyes grew wide with wonder and relief "You really do care, don't you," she decided. A fruitful phase ensued in which Lisi became able to identify anxiety as an "overall prickling" which drove her into inappropriate behavior with men in an attempt to alleviate it. She had previously thought herself "very sexy" because any and all men could make her "prickly." Her improvisations brought the material about her mother to the fore. Deep relaxation exercises combined with stretching and breathing finally allowed her to identify what the body sensations she felt really were. She began to see that men were forever attractive to her because her father had ignored her to please the mother. She tried anything to become close to any man but simultaneously remembered somatically that mother had forbidden access to father.

Lisi is one of many who cannot recognize their body feelings. Many acting-out adolescents, for instance, also suffer from a Borderline Personality Organization. Their frequent relapses into socially unacceptable behavior and the ineffectiveness of present punitive measures have been described by many, without, however, taking into consideration the views stated here.

In clinical practice, one often meets clients who are as plagued by their many symptoms as Lisi and just as unable at first to admit to them. Alissa perhaps exemplifies the Borderline condition best.

Alissa

She was referred after 2 years of combined drug therapy and verbal psychotherapy had kept her from acting-out, but had not been able to induce her to return to school or to do anything but "mope around and hang out." Initially, psychiatric treatment had been ordered for her by a court order after an arrest for soliciting and prostitution. Her upper middle-class parents were profoundly disturbed by their daughter's behavior, and tried repeatedly to shake her out of her torpor after the arrest by offers of jobs, schooling, travel. When the father was first confronted by his daughter's antisocial actions, he flew into an uncontrollable rage and hit her repeatedly. This fact was now used by the daughter as a rationale to refuse all offered aid by her family. However, she voiced no resistance to the suggestion of her psychiatrist to come for dance-movement therapy.

Her mother brought her for the first few sesssions, and anyone unfamiliar with the background would have thought the mother, rather than the daughter, was the patient. While mother wrung her hands, wept, and asked where she might have gone wrong, the daughter comforted her, hugged her, and told her not to worry, she was a fine mother, etc. There was a practiced and somewhat histrionic air about this scene which took place almost immediately upon arrival, as though to impress the therapist with the closeness of the mother-daughter bond. Questioning revealed that the mother was in therapy also, and that Alissa's "troubles" began immediately after a younger, brain-damaged brother had been placed in an institution during Alissa's absence at summer camp, and without her knowledge. The mother claimed "not to have had a minute's trouble" with her daughter before. She described her as moody, charming when it suited her purpose, an erratic student who exasperated her teachers by working just enough to get by, despite strong potential, a rather lonely person who would have "crushes" on either a boy or a girl for a short time and then suddenly drop the new friend

Although all questions were directed to Alissa, she answered none of them, while mother eagerly poured forth volumes of information. Significant in the family's and Alissa's history was the determination with which the younger child's severe disability had been treated. The child was patterned after the Delacato method (1962), with little success. He had also been taken to other specialists all over the United States and abroad, so that all family life was centered almost exclusively around him, until it became apparent that existence outside of a hospital setting would be impossible for him. As the older sister, Alissa had been expected to share the responsibility for the "baby" despite the fact that only four years separated them. The final decision to place the brother, however, was made suddenly and without consulting her.

Alissa's only comment during the first session was that she liked taking care of people and had thought of becoming a Special Education teacher. Through torrents of tears, mother declared that this was "just talk," since Alissa refused to finish her high school requirements.

Alissa herself was an extremely attractive girl with huge eyes, dressed in easygoing, but expensive "hippie" style. She moved slowly, with a floating, ungrounded quality, and had a curious way of stiffening into immobility when looked at. Two sessions per week was agreed upon to which her mother would drive her until the time when Alissa "would get it together enough" to take her driver's test. Apparently, this had become an issue within the family. The parents had agreed to buy Alissa a car if she would get her license and return to school. Alissa, however, had decided that driving a car would add to the pollution of the environment, and made it clear that she expected to be chauffeured. The manipulativeness and inconsistency of these statements were understood by the parents, as was their bribe of a car by Alissa.

The borderline aspects of Alissa's character organization were already visible in the mother's sketch of her daughter's behavior, as well as in the refusal to pollute the environment by driving a car, yet condoning the same pollution if someone else drove it.

Alissa apparently always exhibited contradictory behavior and then rationalized it without being in the least influenced by other people's opinions. What was important to her was to be in control, to manipulate people and things so that she would not have to face her own inadequacies. She appeared adept at simply denying what she didn't want to know. The floating, ungrounded way of gliding rather than walking and the very harmonious, slow sweeping movements were certainly Alissa's own motoric adaptation. The sudden rigidity when she felt looked at also pointed in the direction of borderline features. The psychiatrist had various called her a "preschizophrenic character" and an "as-if" personality. An unreal quality emanated from Alissa and produced a vague countertransferential unease in the therapist. The skill with which she reinforced her mother's guilt by supposedly comforting her while at the same time conveying to the therapist nonverbally that she was not needed because of the intensity of the mother-daughter relationships was awesome. She had induced precisely the emotion people like Alissa know how to produce so well: unease.

As long as the Alissas of this world feel in control, they are able to function well and to figure out, with amazing accuracy, what is expected from them (Deutsch, 1952). This gives their action the ''as if'' quality which belies the concreteness of much of their behavior when they are not in the impulse-ridden phase. Unease was further reinforced when Alissa reported that the psychiatrist whom she had seen for 2 years was a ''fink'' who ''doped her up'' so that she didn't know what she was doing. No attachment to the physician who had treated her for 2 years was visible on the surface. It was agreed that she would stop taking her medication, after this change had been cleared both with the psychiatrist and the parents. It is my conviction, based on 20 years' experience, that people who are heavily medicated benefit only peripherally, if at all, from dance-movement therapy. Amount of dosage and type of drug are important also, of course, and vary considerably in each case. Some drugs, may cause dyskinisia so that the very agency one addresses oneself to, the body Self of the client, is not available, except in diminished form. The effect is similar to verbal therapy with a deaf client (Cain & Cain, 1973; Hall, 1978).

Alissa seemed very pleased by the many telephone conferences that were necessary to free her from her prescriptions. As a ''reward'' to the therapist she agreed to participate in movement. An interpretation that she perhaps was treating her therapist as she would like to be treated herself was met with a sneer in her angelic face. She thought the telephone calls were a sign that she had controlled the therapist psychically into sharing her supposed wish for freedom from medication. She began to revile both her former psychiatrist and her parents as old-fashioned and rigid, and requested three sessions per week instead of the agreed-upon two. This request was refused because the wish to form a collusive alliance against the important people in her life looked like yet another manipulation which could not possibly produce growth. This event occurred very early in the treatment.

After all the verbalizations, arrangements, and setting of boundaries—an indispensable phase, if the course of intervention was to succeed—therapy proper now began.

True to her promise, Alissa "danced." Attired in embroidered Indian gowns, a flower in her long curly hair, she would glide into the room and trace its circumference with slow, measured steps. Sometimes, she would strike a pose, arms stretched to both sides, head thrown back and then resume her pacing. On occasion she would hum tuneless songs that accelerated into loud, deep calls without words. When she became aware of the therapist watching her, she would stand still, smile, and indicate with harmonious gesturing that she was issuing an invitation to join her. She met refusal of the invitation with equanimity, but attempts to investigate the meaning of her rite or to change it were simply ignored. A feeling connection between Alissa and her therapist arose nevertheless as Alissa continued to present her ritual dance.

The therapist's countertransferential unease now began to give way to pictures of Alissa as a reincarnation of Isadora Duncan. Self-analysis revealed this to be a reflection of Alissa's omnipotence and prepared the therapist somewhat for the next event. Some 3 months after the biweekly ritual dances, Alissa appeared in jeans and big leather boots, high on marijuana, waving her new driver's license about. She had brought a new reggae record with her and began a triumphal dance expressing ecstasy, sexual arousal, and the unmistakable wish to impress. Strutting and cavorting, she cynically asked if she would be discharged now since she had "got it together," and received her driver's license and was prepared to return to school to fulfill the few missing requirements for her diploma. Recognizing the shift in her behavior, but also aware that this was the other face of the same control issue that had been skirted before, the therapist asked how the effect of the marijuana high differed from that of the drugs she had to take previously. "It's the same, you old cow,'' the ex-Isadora exclaimed. ''Bet you haven't screwed a man in ten years.''

Here, finally was an allusion to the behavior that had brought her into conflict with the law. The effect of the marijuana seemed a symbolic bridge to the ''fink of a psychiatrist'' who had kept her under control. This therapist's more neutral stance and the often voiced assumption that Alissa could ''get it together'' if she wanted to were partially responsible for the swing. More importantly, Alissa accusingly screamed that she was tired of all that slow dance stuff, especially when the therapist was so stupid as to fail to recognize a medieval chanting and court ritual when she saw it. Acknowledging her disappointment, the therapist told her that she had no magic, but needed words as well as movement for communication. She was also asked to abstain from smoking before and during her sessions. ''You don't give a shit about me, do you?'' Alissa yelled, and wanted to leave. The information that she was expected to finish her hour had a strongly quieting effect. Grumbling, she removed her boots and began to prod the therapist gently with her feet, obviously an invitation to join the dance.

Alissa's manifold symbolic actions in this hour made it clear that much of her difficulty had been brought to the surface by simply accepting her dances. But how to interpret, under stand, integrate, so much material to a person whose foremost aim is to stay ''boss'' at all cost?

Alissa had begun to understand that it would be hard to manipulate her therapist and that much was known about her despite her denials. Perhaps the outburst had adaptational purposes. Also, she had at least peripherally mentioned sexual matters, though projected onto the therapist (Friedman, 1969).

This new raucous Alissa proved herself a fine dancer who could easily follow any and all instructions, and was so enthusiastic about dancing and movement in general that she wrote to various dance departments for admissions.

During this time, the sessions looked like dance classes. *Plies* and *releves* were corrected. Alissa learned to center herself and used breathing exercises. She no longer wanted to improvise, but strove for a dancer's physical agility. Her need to build a different body and self image was acknowledged verbally. But this interpretation glanced off Alissa as though she were a glacier. She thought she wanted to learn body mechanics and dance techniques, period. She told the therapist defiantly that she was free to read anything into her actions.

In the meantime, her parents were pleased, high school was a "cinch," and only the therapist was back with her previous unease. During the session, which always began with a warm-up, all of Alissa's movements seemed to begin and end in the same place. They stayed concrete. She said they did not evoke anything other than the immediate muscle sensation of "doing." There was no joy in the movement itself, no exploration of new planes or space, just a dogged pursuit of more and more difficult exercises, structured dances and combinations. Conspicuous also was her inability to combine breathing patterns appropriately with the executed rhythms. Most sessions ended with a wild spurt of energetic spinning or jumping at high speed.

Alissa began to read dance publications, became an expert in anatomy, and began to fantasize about becoming a dance therapist herself. She still angrily warded off investigation of the initial outburst that ushered in this phase. Attempts to deal with the covert negative transference were also pushed aside. Joylessness, cynicism, and mechanical aping of the therapist's movements were very much in evidence.

Speculations about Alissa's past had to remain just that because she warded off all questioning, and denied and suppressed feelings aroused by the sessions. Nonetheless it can be postulated that the depressions, guilt, and frantic activity with which Alissa's mother surrounded her son prevented her from helping the little girl to integrate opposing feeling states. The brief moments in which the parents' full attention shone onto Alissa's life, alternating with their total unavailability when immersed in helping their son, more likely than not reinforced Alissa's perception of the world as cut into two unconnected halves, one filled with loving parents, the other with emotionally unavailable giants who moved other people's limbs about as in the brother's patterning. The father's propensity toward un-controlled rage was probably also a factor in reinforcing the small Alissa's perceptions of one person being really two strangers.

During the last half of her senior year in high school, Alissa became a model citizen indeed. She volunteered some time at a school for special children, took dancing lessons, and appeared punctually for her sessions. However, there was no talk of add-ing a third session now. The hours were filled with attempts to stretch further, contract more correctly, turn out more widely, and to use dance therapy jargon picked up during workshops with other dance therapists. Alissa was accepted at a prestigious college where the openness of the structure would allow her to continue efforts toward becoming a dance therapist.

Warnings that Alissa was not yet ready to leave her present protected structured life went unheeded by her parents and herself. Off she went in a cloud of triumphant control.

Just before Christmas holiday break she was back, wide-eyed, depressed, and with a new set of symptoms. During choir practice in a church off campus, while singing a hymn, she had suddenly felt transparent. She claimed she could see her own veins and heart with the blood coursing through them. Her flesh had become waxen, flexible, and "illuminated." At the same time, she had seen a vision of the Virgin Mary. Peace flooded her and she was determined to convert to the Catholic faith. Appraised of this, her parents brought her home. Because of their own ethnic, but not religious, identification with Judaism, the threatened conversion appeared almost as bad to them as the arrest 4 years ago.

The therapist agreed to see Alissa daily and to "get her back in shape" for the start of the next semester although declining to accept this deadline. Crisis-intervention never-theless seemed appropriate in view of Alissa's delusions.

The Isadora Duncan-like performances began again, this time with sound effects. Alissa had unearthed a record of sitar music to which she now danced. The sounds swept her into a hypnotic twilight state during which she lost her fear of being looked at, which she had never verbalized but always acted upon. She engaged in autoerotic activity in the form of wetting her underpants slightly, giggling, stopping the flow of urine just in time, and then running to the toilet during the session.

The therapist responded to this need for both toilet training and approval by mother and direct gratification by saying: "I am glad you can wait to reach the toilet."

After these episodes, Alissa's general behavior became more primitive during the sessions. She had a need to skip to polka music, sway to waltzes, play hop scotch, or simply to run around in a circle. Every once in a while she would stop smilingly to be admired. Finally, a true regression to the fixation point had been achieved. Alissa began to act like a mischievous toddler testing her mother's tolerance. This "toddler-phase" is a regularly occurring event in the successful treatment of Borderline Personality Organization. Hide-and-seek became a favorite game. Her daily arrival was marked by joyous excitement. The therapist felt she was in the presence of a warm, emerging human being. Body contact was shunned because Alissa was convinced that her skin would retain indentations from a hug, and become "illuminated" again. She began to read the *Confessions of St. Augustine*, and to compare herself to this Saint and his life. She ignored assurances that past mistakes did not need to be atoned by a saintly life.

Alissa now began to compose and to write it down in Old English script using a calligraphic pen. The first letter on each page was illuminated as in medieval manuscripts. She accepted an interpretation that she possibly was symbolically illuminating letters instead of her skin.

Just before the beginning of the semester, Alissa announced that she would not return to school. Crushed and angry , her parents withdrew Alissa from treatment. Not yet strong enough to insist on continuance herself, Alissa began to send her lovely poems to the therapist by mail. Approximately a year later, she telephoned to say that she was joining a commune in which healing by laying on of hands and by herbs was practiced.

Another year passed before she appeared again for sessions, brought by her mother. In the commune, a young man experienced a revelation of himself as the Second Coming of Christ, and sought twelve female apostles to follow him. Alissa was to be number three, with initiation consisting of intercourse with the young man in the presence of the other apostles-to-be. Immediately after this "initiation," Alissa underwent a recurrence of all her symptoms including the vision of the Virgin Mary and her own physical transparency. However, she had enough strength to call her parents, who immediately flew to the distant state where the commune was located, and brought her home.

In treatment for the third time, Alissa settled down to an in-depth intervention. She jokingly began to call the therapist "Mrs. Rock," because "she never fell apart." Intervention in the form of Effort-Shape based exploration became possible since a true therapeutic alliance had finally been formed (Friedman, 1969). Alissa's ego could now tolerate and even welcome as valuable, work on body fundamentals and conscious examination of her flow qualities. She began to build a new body image and formed a more cohesive self. Eventually, she entered a school for Hebrew Teachers, and there immersed herself in a course of studies of her own heritage. Though many of the mystic qualities of her psyche were reinforced by prayer and ritual there, her parents were able to accept her otherworldliness in this frame of reference.

The latest crisis came on the eve of her wedding to a young member of her religious community. The fear of receiving permanent indentations in her skin was revived, as was the wish to become a saint who is removed from the "blemish" of physical life. The fears subsided on accepting the realities of marital life.

Alissa is now a young wife earnestly striving to reconcile what she has learned about herself in therapy, with the demands of her life. Still fragile, her ability to sublimate is increasing. Her strong need for physical tension release has been translated into leading an Israeli folk-dancing group, and some of her poems have been published. The need for communal sharing, and the family life she never had is being met by her devotion to her temple. Most importantly, she has learned to read her own body signals accurately, and can thus forestall regression and pathologic splitting.

In summary, it can be stated that Alissa's ability for reality testing remained unimpaired through her many crises, though her ability to *experience* reality was often severely distorted by the oscillation of contradictory feelings about her self. The capacity to establish true object relationships was severely impaired due to the mechanism of splitting, until a combination of educational and therapeutic measures helped to establish a transferential relationship which could grow organically without her manipulative control. Dance Movement Therapy was the intervention of choice for her because it offers tension discharge, body-image building, strengthening of body boundaries, and the possibility of integrating diffuse and diverse instinctual manifestations nonverbally, despite the presence of splitting and denial of affect.

More specifically, dance-movement therapy provided a place where Alissa could express her fantasies through movement when verbalization seemed too frightening. She could fantasize herself beloved and understood by the therapist, like an infant who imagines that her mother feels what she feels and knows what she knows. This paved the way for testing and aping the therapist in angry rebellion, another steppingstone she had not negotiated fully with her parents. They, after all, had been preoccupied with her disabled sibling. Alissa's strong agression almost forced a premature separation, but work on body placement and movement during sessions always drained off the excess tension and gave her the opportunity to build a different and firmer body image. Concomitantly, her ability to trust an important other-than-self grew sufficiently to overcome her narcissistic wounds, permitting her to go and to come back as the need arose.

***

Obsession, Compulsion, and Movement

The people whose dance-movement therapy treatment has been described thus far were all not classically analyzable, as the expression goes. But according to psychoanalytic theory, Raymond, Cassie, and many others certainly were. They suffered from obsessions and compulsions.

I had long thought such clients would do well in dance-movement therapy because the very agencies to which psychoanalysis addresses itself, thinking and talking, are deeply affected in obsession compulsion. In this flight from feelings, obsessive-compulsive people go back to the time in life when words had an almost magic quality. When they first learned to say "cookie," mother might have been so pleased she gave them one immediately; when they began to express other things with the correct word, the pleasure of people around them reinforced their conviction that words are something very special that have the quality of evoking special effects. Words open new doors of perception and mastery for the growing child. As life goes on, words and speech lose some of their magic quality. Language becomes a function one uses without really giving it any distinct emotional quality. It is a safe activity insofar as one can choose one's words carefully and either speak volumes or withhold them altogether. Normally, one is in control of what one says. But for the obsessive-compulsive person, words lose this practical, everyday value. In their avoidance of any feeling connections to the world, they reinvest words and language with the magic power they once had in infancy (Fenichel, 1945). The analyst in such cases is confronted by an analysand who must be treated through impaired functions and channels. Therefore, dance-movement therapy offers a more direct and less obstructed route toward better functioning for such clients.

In the classically obsessive personality, behavior and thoughts continue long after voluntary action has taken care of their aim. Closure is never really achieved.

My client Cassie, for instance, did all her homework in minutest detail and to perfection. But at bedtime she began to doubt that she had done it at all and regularly kept herself from sleep by getting up and checking what she had done over and over again. When her mother insisted that she stay in bed, she did so, but at the huge price of insomnia. During such a sleepless night, the thought came to her: I would like to kill my mother. It's really her fault I can't sleep.

Beset by such frightening thought-wishes, Cassie was nevertheless calm. Her feelings simply did not connect with her thoughts. During treatment she reassured me, and herself, by saying: "I wouldn't really kill my mother. The next thing that would happen is that my father would keep me from sleeping instead." The callousness and grandiosity in this thought hardly need be pointed out. Such cruel thoughts are present in many people whose lives have forced them into the creation of obsessional symptoms. But because they cannot allow the feelings that connected to such fantasies to erupt, they often experience physiologic distress instead of anxiety.

Cassie suffered from headaches and constipation. The tragedy for people like Cassie consists in the fact that they may, after a while in treatment, gather insight into the illogical and destructive nature of some of their thoughts and actions, but this does not change their behavior. Their obsessions are "persistent, intellectualized thought patterns while their compulsions are persistent, ritualized behavior patterns" (Salzman, 1977).

When Cassie obeyed her mother and stayed in bed instead of checking her work over for the hundredth time, her anxiety merely intensified until she had to think "I want to kill my mother." She could not allow herself to think that she had really complied with all demands. Of course such obsessive ruminations were insufferable for a child who was also obedient, dependable, intellectually superior, and a perfectionist. She had to atone for her awful obsessional thoughts by getting headaches and by being constipated. When her mother took her to a physician to correct the constipation which would not yield to medication, Cassie's murderous thoughts increased in intensity. Defecating normally meant losing control over her natural body functions and over her thoughts. Perhaps if she defecated freely, she would also say freely: I want to kill mother. She had to stay defended and held in at all costs.

In this struggle for control, she became a pale wraithlike child, the proverbial little ''old soul'' who read and played by herself and rationalized her isolation as superiority over the other rougher, rowdier children she was forced to go to school with. Although she fantasized herself to be a dancer and gymnast of talent, Cassie was encumbered by the physical armor Reich (1949) describes so well. Her feelings had been denied access to their motoric expression for so long that she was rigid and sometimes subject to painful spasms in her legs. It was as though she unconsciously fortified her whole physical being against the intrustion of more and more alien thoughts.

Cassie presented the typical picture of someone for whom repression has not worked sufficiently. Too much stayed in her consciousness, and only by keeping feelings separate from her thoughts could she exist without disintegrating entirely under the weight of her morbid fantasies. But Cassie was a child whose difficulties had not persisted long. Therapeutic interaction was fruitful once her motility was tapped in the service of expression. Her treatment did not last as long as that of adults who presented themselves with obsessive systems of long standing. Among them, the difficulties engendered by obsessive thinking and ritualistic behavior were most poignantly and completely incorporated by Raymond.

Raymond

Raymond was referred to dance-movement therapy after a year of competent psychoanalytic intervention had nevertheless produced so many doubtful ruminations and resentments in him that his analysis had ground to a halt. His wife had left him, ostensibly because his compulsive behavior had taken over so much of his life that he had to work at home and could no longer follow his profession. The rituals which kept him psychologically safe took up so much of his time that the usual family and work activities had been truncated. Raymond had been trained as an accountant. He was the third of five children in a family that prided itself on its tradition and puritanical heritage. Raymond, according to his mother, had "all the advantages." He went to a prestigious prep school and to an even more prestigious college. He was a fine athlete, and up to the time of his marriage, had given every promise of following in the footsteps of his forebears. By the time he presented himself for dance-movement therapy not much of his heritage and gentle upbringing was visible.

His scant blond hair was tousled above a high forehead that was worriedly wrinkled. Breathing heavily, and wearing a strange combination of clothes that looked borrowed, he stayed put in the doorway for some moments in order to check that "he had everything." This ritual of checking all his pockets took place even before he introduced himself. It was to stay with him throughout a year of biweekly visits. Although we didn't specifically analyze the meaning of this particular ritual, it disappeared when Raymond felt more certain that all his body parts and belongings were realistically under control.

The first thing he wanted his new therapist to know was that he wished to be in therapy with her because her intervention had to do with the body. He had had enough of all this talking stuff which, he suspected, had influenced him adversely so that now he had lost his wife. Exhausted from his tirade but also satisfied that he had let the therapist know the things most important to him, he leaned back and studied her intently. With something resembling the air of a schoolmaster, he then began an interrogation. Could the therapist really move well and where had she gone to school? And how had she managed to impress his ex-analyst with her worth and value since clearly her type of intervention was most unorthodox? It turned out that in Raymond's opinion his ex-analyst wasn't any good, but that still made him better by a long shot than this therapist.

In the meantime Raymond revealed himself as not particularly clean, his fingernails bore evidence of having been chewed, and he comported himself with the portentous dignity of an elder statesman. Head held erect above muscular shoulders, he bowed toward the therapist in a courtly manner whenever his questions reached a point that could be interpreted as arrogant. The therapist told him that her training could readily be ascertained from the diplomas in the waiting room and that she could understand his concern about starting therapy with someone like herself. He immediately wilted and asked what he should do. Before the answer could be given, he remarked that he enjoyed social dancing enormously, and that at school he had been a member of the gymnastics team. Asked if he felt like performing some of the calisthenics that must have been part of his training, he declined, explaining that the surroundings of the studio were not conducive to such activity. He was, however, willing to walk around and to examine the collection of records. He had taken off his ill-fitting long coat under which he wore greasy black pants and an ancient green sweater with holes in the elbows. Under this was a shirt of nondescript color with a torn collar. Heavy gold cufflinks dangled precariously in the worn buttonholes of his sleeves and his foodstained cravate was adorned by a stickpin that must have been an heirloom. What was one to make of this splendid scarecrow?

He put on a jazz record, opened his arms awkwardly to the sides and slowly swayed from side to side in time with the syncopated and complex music. It was difficult to understand how he managed to execute this swaying. His entire body stayed stiff and overly controlled with little movement in any of his joints. It seemed more as though he were giving himself tight little pushes from side to side. When his performance ended he asked for an interpretation of his movements. He had heard that all movement means something. The therapist told him that eventually they would discover together what these things meant to him, but that right now, she didn't know either. She told him she had observed that he didn't look very comfortable, but that this could be a reflection of being there for the first time and not knowing her very well.

Raymond's answering comment was of the kind he would

use repeatedly. "Oh well," he said, "I guess you don't know too much either, do you." Then he asked for the therapist's card since he seemed to have mislaid the one his former analyst had given him, and cancelled the next session. It seems he "had something to do that day." He was told that of course he was free to cancel but that if he wished to be this therapist's client there were certain minimal rules, one of them being that cancelled sessions had to be made up at a convenient time for both and that these sessions had to be paid for whether he could "find the time" to make up or not. Raymond made a startling response. Just in case, he needed a second one of the business cards for his hip pocket, and he thought he could make it to the next session after all.

Over the next few months, Raymond revealed a great deal about the etiology of his erratic behavior. Apparently the turning point in his life had been his marriage. A lonely young man, full of anxieties and secret yearning for unattainable honors, for orgies and occult sects, he was overwhelmed but gratified when he met his future wife. She was a popular girl who decided to go after him because "nobody else could get him." They met at school where up to that point he had been a loner who excelled at his studies and was an excellent gymnast. His father had recently died and on his deathbed had enjoined Raymond to "take care of mother." Raymond took his request literally and tried to move back into his mother's house after having lived either in boarding school or at college since he was twelve. Mother, however, wanted none of this. She begged him to devote himself to his studies and to make a man of himself. Raymond went back to school, wrote daily letters to his mother and dreamed himself even more deeply into his secret world until Bette came along. He claimed that she seduced him, teasing him about "wasting his wonderful penis." Raymond thought that she was quite right. He was unusually well endowed and had always held a grudge against girls for not recognizing his superiority. Even at boarding school, he had never been able to obtain a steady date or a dancing partner. He was odd, but superior, according to himself.

His view of himself exhibited all the earmarks of ambivalence. With omnipotent grandiosity,he thought himself better than others, but he expected those inferior others to accept his specialness without any effort on his part to acquaint them with his gifts. He thought they should know who he was from his name and from his performance at school. In then current jargon, "laid back" might be a good description of how Raymond presented himself. But under his blase worldliness, there was just a little too much passivity, and under grandiose claims of special gifts, just a little too much insecurity. Raymond, like other obsessive people, had to be in control, and had to rationalize everything. He appeared utterly devoted to his mother and sister. But he also spoke derisively of them as mere women. The ambivalence in all his undertakings and interpersonal relationships was marked. His wife was wonderful while with him, but a whore who had left him. His analyst was great, but not great enough for him. This therapist was barely in the running at all, a mere ex-dancer who had made it into therapy as a professional, he didn't know how. In the meantime, Raymond had difficulty in such simple exercises as letting his head hang down on his chest. He simply couldn't bend that stiff neck enough to just let his chin touch his chest. If he managed to get his head down at all, he would immediately screw up his eyes and ask if this was far enough down.

Eventually, a warm-up was found that satisfied him. He would march in, stop at the door for his ritualistic checking of all pockets and then throw himself into a series of pushups and sit-ups as though he were training for the Olympics. His biceps and thighs always quivered right from the start when he did these exercises, not only when he was tired, but he never seemed to notice this. Apparently invigorated, he would then ask for music, preferably ballet music. Raymond had decided that he would now master the art of ballet. But while he could hold a *relevé* for many counts and even do something that resembled a plie, he simply couldn't bow in a *reverence*, roll up from it, or bend backward. He substituted grand, sweeping arm motions. It was as though he could move arms and legs in order to connect him with the rest of his body, but his body was rigid.

A series of breathing exercise was instituted. Raymond could breathe deeply indeed. So deeply, as a matter of fact, that he hyperventilated and blacked out. Of course he had an explanation for this, also. He had learned Yoga earlier but was now out of practice, hence the hyperventilation. Raymond did not want to examine why he had so purposefully hyperventilated. According to him, talking about things and situations had spoiled his analysis and he wasn't about to let the same thing happen in this therapy. This statement was a sign that a positive attachment was beginning to form underneath Raymond's negativism. This thought was shared with him. Instead of answering, he presented the therapist with his first dream. Raymond dreamed that he took the hand of a woman in front of a huge auditorium full of people. Immediately afterward, there was an explosion.

Raymond didn't want to talk about his dream either, but he was willing to illustrate it through movement. Explaining carefully that he was taking the therapist by the hand only because she happened to be in the same room with him, he grabbed her and took her around the studio. Sometimes he would stand stock-still and point into a corner. Then he flung her aside and himself on the floor in illustration of the explosion. All this was executed with the most detached air possible. Once again, he wanted an interpretation without venturing any opinion or association of his own. After brooding about the therapist's statement that she could see how distressed about and suspicious of verbal interaction he was, Raymond decided to demonstrate that all that had been said was wrong. He insisted that his dream meant that if he really committed himself to the therapeutic venture, the same thing would happen with the therapist that had happened with his wife; she would betray him, that was what the explosion signified. As a matter of fact, he thought all therapists of all persuasions were unreliable because their services were for sale and not freely given.

This sounded like a statement about competition with siblings and about the unhappy turn of events with his wife, possibly even about something that might have happened to him in the past with his mother. An explosion after contact with a woman pointed to fear of intimate contact with females, to castration, and possible annihilation fears in connection with body disintegration fantasies. Was Raymond a latent homosexual or a Borderline personality? But he had pushed the therapist aside when the imaginary explosion was about to occur in his "improvisation." Did Raymond wish to protect the therapist? Was he looking for assurance that she would not leave him as his wife had left him? He called her a whore. Did that mean therapists who accepted money for their services were whores in his internal constellation? Were therapists and whore equated inside of him to mean: the therapist as transference object receives the feelings produced by the departing wife? No wonder, then, that he didn't want to see the therapist as a professional but as someone who should be controllable by his demands. However, the relationship was still too tenuous to bear the brunt of such strong currents openly. The therapist told Raymond that it looked to her as though something in their relationship might have become important enough to him to make him speculate whether therapists were trustworthy. In response, Raymond began to perspire heavily. But, as with his other actions, he did not acknowledge this. He was conspicuously split off from reading and truly feeling all his body feelings. Instead, he departed with a derisive sneer.

When Raymond next appeared, he had thought of a different approach strategy, one that characterized his mode of conducting himself in the sessions for several months. He began to make sarcastic remarks about everything that went on during therapy. As he once again checked his belongings during his entrance ritual, he commented that the therapist looked like a warden who was cataloging a prisoner's belongings; when he did his warm-up, she reminded him of a coach who had been an unmerciful slave driver; at the barre, he found her an "excruciatingly stuck-up ballet mistress"; when he improvised to his beloved jazz record, and she did not join him, she became one of the women who apparently rejected his advances regularly.

While he appeared to relish any and all movement experiences, there was always a caustic comment about how harsh he thought the therapist and how harshly others had treated him. He told of being sent to a kindergarten when he was two and a half so "his mother could attend to business." It turned out that much of the family's income then was earned by his mother's involvement with high fashion industries while his father pursued scholarly interests that didn't bring any monetary rewards. Raymond somehow could only focus on the "betrayal" of his mother in leaving the children with servants and sending them to school. But while he was able to tell about these events, there was still a conspicuous absence of any somatically felt sense connected to these happenings. Raymond remained sarcastic and preferred to distance himself from his own life experience.

Conspicuous also was the mode in which he chose to relate all this . He never talked if he was sitting still. His life history was told as he was moving or dancing. It was as though his motor drive would not let him be still and reflect. Instead, it forced him into motor activity that was often not at all connected to what he was saying. The fact that his anxiety and the need to move was aroused by his recollections was dealt with by any exercise Raymond liked or had learned in the past. He had allowed balletic exercises to be introduced at the barre because he thought it would make him more graceful. He experienced his athlete's bulging muscles as unattractive and his bound, heavy way of moving as "klutzy." His improvisations also were always awkward and lacked fluidity. He experienced a small improvement in his ability to relax and breathe deeply without losing himself when doing Yogic breathing *assanahs*. At the same time he told about being left with a variety of nurses and governesses before being sent to boarding school.

Raymond's voice became low and he averted his gaze when he spoke of the women who had taken care of him. He invariably began to fiddle with his clothing when the subject came up. The therapist noted aloud that perhaps he found it difficult now to make relationships with women because his mother, the nurses, and his wife had all left him. For the first time, Raymond was able to respond with his total being after this interpretation. Crying quietly, he crossed his arms over his chest, sat down and rocked himself rhythmically in time to his own sobs. With deep sadness, he spoke of wrapping himself into his mother's velvet robe in order to recapture her essence during her absence. He also remembered entertaining himself by imagining that irridescent bubbles would come out of the skies, envelop him and transport him to his mother. At other times, he would hide behind the heavy draperies of the family's dining room while they were entertaining until the dust there made him sneeze. He was ignonimiously dragged out into the light to be "pawed" by the laughing company. He thought that it was then that he had learned both to be sarcastic and aloof—sarcastic like the guests who said: "Look at that little boy. Why isn't he in bed?" and aloof like his mother who curtly ordered the nurse to put him to bed so that he wouldn't disturb the assemblage any more. After that, he became shy and tongue-tied in the presence of strangers. He confided that the same shyness now still overcame him when in the presence of "young ladies or prospective employers."

The painful subject of his lack of employment now arose. He simply could not bring himself to follow up on opportunities for positions arranged for by his family. By now he had moved his handiman's shop into a stable on the family's estate and existed there in "splendid isolation" in the former groom's small apartment. Customers rarely found their way there so that Raymond was soon left without funds. He improvised an air-tight stove which unfortunately collapsed and nearly burned him.

Throughout all these tribulations, he paid his fees regularly, though never without an accusing speech and a detailed account of how he had obtained the money through lawn-mowing, chauffeuring his mother's friends, and other odd jobs.

His latest fantasy was that he would become some rich lady's gigolo so that he could pay more than the therapist's fee. He had begun to enjoy his sessions and even looked forward to them. He was now working on both floor stretches and on stretches at the barre because he complained of feeling "cramped and locked." He reported regularly being flooded with relief when his right muscles were able to give in temporarily. He called it "muscles letting go their stranglehold." He also managed to place his hand as close to the therapist's as possible but always pulled it back quickly if there was danger of accidentally touching.

His improvisations took on a different quality. He began to dance in half *relevé* and with slightly bent knees so that all his movements took on a springy air. His musical selections also changed. He now favored country style music in which poor country boys either lost their "purty country gals" or were jilted by hardhearted women. He usually sang along in twangy, nasal tones but with lots of gusto. He invited the therapist to dance and sing along. When she declined, he made certain that he placed himself in such a position that she could not miss the slightest one of his movements. Quite obviously, and appropriately, she had become the object on which he hung his oedipal longings.

Before this was interpretted, yet another change took place. Raymond was offered a job by a former college mate who had also been left by his wife. Raymond was to be a financial consultant for the clients of a well-known law firm. As a result, Raymond's insecurities surfaced and hit him with all their force. He forgot his training as an accountant and his previous experience with stocks and bonds. Gone also was the playful, ineptly seductive country playboy of previous sessions. Instead, an ashen-faced young man appeared who needed to "check himself out" several times each hour, who reeked of anxiety sweat and was unable to take showers. This phobic response had to do with the fact that one needs to take one's clothes off when bathing and Raymond suddenly found the sight of his own body distasteful. Stretches no longer gave him relief. Instead, he wanted to pound the floor with his fists and then with his head. There was something so penitential in these actions that he was asked if by chance he felt he had to atone for something. He gave one of his scornful glances. Of course, how could the therapist be so stupid? he wanted to know. Who could like someone who had just wanted to be a gigolo? It was bad enough that the therapist knew about that. How would his future employers feel about him if they found out? It was argued at length that nobody could guess his thought unless he spoke of them. At this point, Raymond remembered his extensive reading. Could it be, he asked, that he really had wanted to sleep with his mother?—that the gigolo fantasy and the subsequent atonement rite really had to do with incest?

He looked at the therapist, turned scarlet, and suddenly realized that he must have directed some of these incestuous feelings at her as well. But he recovered quickly enough. "That's what you get paid for, isn't it?" he concluded, with all of his former arrogance back in place. Then he dropped the entire subject and discussed which one of his ancient but well-cut blazers he should wear to his interview.

His sudden, if transient, insight was encouraging because despite the relief he gained during sessions, Raymond still seemed too caught up in magic and ritual to be able to hold a job. He couldn't even enjoy his own fantasies. His overstrict superego saw to that. He was also still isolated from family and friends, criticizing them from afar and surfacing only long enough on weekends to be ridiculed for his advances to "young ladies."

However, in spite of the therapist's silent formulations to the contrary, Raymond had taken in a certain amount of gratification through the motor activities that were connected to her as the "good enough object." This was brought home when several agitated telephone calls later he reappeared, this time employed and sporting a haircut that shaped his hair like a bowl around his face. Before going to his interview, he had visited his brother who had insisted that he take a bath. When he refused to go to a barber as well, brother had simply taken the scissors and "fixed him up." Raymond then explained that he hadn't bathed before because the cold water in his stable apartment didn't take any of the odors away. Here was the curious ambivalence again. Yes, Raymond could take in good feelings, he could perceive reality and was beginning to recapture both memories and body feelings; but he still had to undo and deny what had been achieved by unusual rationalizations and phobic behavior.

What kept him going through these rough spots was the memory of physical relaxation and feeling good after movement experiences.

With Raymond's employment, a new phase was ushered in. He discovered that some of his co-workers liked him and wanted to take him under their wing. He was extremely suspicious of this because some of them belonged to his ex-wife's "old set." He thought that they might be messengers in her service and that she wanted him back even though he had convinced himself that all women were "no good." He often ventured his opinion but always took it back with a courtly bow in the therapist's direction, saying, "Present company excepted." Suspicious Raymond nontheless began to prepare himself for a possible meeting with his former wife by practicing all the latest rock and roll fads. He wanted to impress her with his sophistication and not foster any notion in her mind for doubt that he might be missing her. He wanted to appear debonair and worldly. In these new dances, he found himself to be entirely out of breath in a short while. Again breathing exercises were instituted to allay these anxiety attacks.

This time, the result was very different. Raymond assumed the *Sleeping Child Assanah,* which resembles the fetal position, while kneeling. Gently, he rocked himself forward and back, forward and back, moaning softly to himself. Slowly, words formed. "Alone, all alone," he sang, "all alone I play by myself." He sat up and showed how he used to play with cars and build roads for them. "Mother's gone," he sang, "brother's gone, I will play." Suddenly, his soft song gave way to laughter. Raymond made his imaginary cars crash into each other. Exultantly, he turned to the therapist, "I made them all disappear in a car crash. I killed my mother, my father, everyone, for leaving me. And maybe I'll kill you too—no, don't worry, people like me don't kill people like you."

At this point, the therapist was glad that Raymond wanted to reassure her because his recreation carried the conviction of reality. An interpretation was offered that referred back to the dream in which a woman and an explosion had been the main elements. Raymond looked sheepish, then said that he "felt good" because the therapist had been able "to pull it all together."

It was also noted that Raymond's movements had taken on the fluidity and postural involvement missing otherwise during his memory recall. At least during this moment, his body and mind had been unified and expressed fully and interdependently material that pressed for discharge. That Raymond was angry, hurt, and vengeful was clear. That he could not tolerate his own feelfings and had to disavow them or punish himself for them was equally clear. Yet he still did not like to reflect upon his feelings, nor did he try to free-associate verbally. His improvisations and sudden spurts of self-knowledge burst upon him with little warning, usually as the result of relaxation techniques and breathing exercises. He rarely wanted to work through what he discovered. But this time Raymond was so fascinated by his experience of an imaginary car crash that he was drawn back to it again and again. It was as though he were looking for a missing piece. He never again relived the episode of what might have been a recovered childhood fantasy with as much intensity as the first time, yet he tried to stage the incident repeatedly and managed to add a description of the room in which it had taken place and of the nurse then in charge of him.

The recovery of the childhood game and fantasy was recognized as "screen memory" because there was something too pat and condensed about the entire episode. Was it fury at his ex-wife that had precipitated this event or anxiety about thought-murders committed long ago? Greenson (1958) has defined the acting out of past experience as screen memories. He is convinced that the acting out distorts the recall by providing wish fulfillment and tension release. Nevertheless, he also sees the nonverbal communication as a reaching out toward an important person, in this case, the therapist for whom the memory was enacted. For Greenson, and other analysts, all acting in the sessions is a resistance against speech. But dance-movement therapists hypothesize that the residue of all life's experiences are stored in the body and can be recovered under appropriate circumstances. The need to finish past conflict in the present has also been discussed. Why then did Raymond have to go back to this apparently complete piece of life history, why could he not finish it? Freud (1905) said a long time ago that we act what we cannot think. Whose theory then was to yield the correct answer to Raymond's dilemma?

As it turned out, psychoanalytic theory and dance-movement therapy theory were both right. Raymond's memory recall was not complete and could be construed as a screen memory, but it also opened the door for the recovery of trauma that, to begin with, was too abhorrent to Raymond to acknowledge.

As he ruminated once again upon his early abandonment and played out the car game he fiddled with his clothing as he had done previously when talking about his nurses. He said he felt uncomfortable, too warm, fidgety. Slowly the familiar reek of his anxiety began to fill the room. He started to pace, and asked for one of his country records. As usual, he would dance instead of talk, about what shackled him to the past. He spread his arms in the gesture the therapist knew well by now, threw his head back and slightly to the side, and placed one foot in front of the other. Looking like Christ on the Cross, his pelvis began to thrust spasmodically. He held this pose for some moments, than shrank toward the floor. The memories came in a flood.

One of the nurses had bathed him every night and shown him how to masturbate. Later, he was allowed to sleep in her bed when frightened and she had encouraged him to masturbate in her presence. The little boy had not known what felt more delicious to him: the sensations in his genitals, or the warmth of the nurse's bed, or the fact that she had given him the gift of self-pleasuring. When she left, he blamed himself, convinced that he driven her away by not masturbating enough for her. He resolved that he would never touch himself again and to become a saint. He had kept his word until he married. His ex-wife, too, enjoyed it if he stroked his penis into erection. He often did so to please her, but in doing so he broke his secret vow to the nurse. He became less and less potent and had to resort to more and more rituals to keep functioning.

The interaction with Raymond became more and more verbal after this pivotal happening. The tensions and crampings, strange rituals, and compulsive behavior no longer obstructed Raymond's associative flow. He began to create dances in which the mourning for his early abandonment and the death of his father were expressed. With characteristic grandiosity, he chose the *Funeral March* from *Aida* as his accompaniment.

The ritual of "checking himself" ceased. He began to talk of what the functions of the ritual had been. He said they reassured him that he had "not lost anything." i.e., and his ex-wife, nor his nurse had not taken his penis from him.

Soon thereafter, Raymond met a "lady" with whom he formed a lasting attachment. He also volunteered his services to his local recreation department where he began to give Yoga lessons.

When his need for companionship and his strong motor drive had been fulfilled, his therapy moved into almost exclusively verbal channels where the particulars of his many fantasies and phobias could be explored in detail.

This is a regularly occurring fact: when the motor drive is tamed, free associations flow, and the split between body and mind can be healed.

All the people whose cases have been presented here needed to find access to their motor drive. The reason for this was multiply determined. For those fixated in the oral stage, it became essential to dissolve the barriers of developmental arrests. They had to build, or rebuild, body images. All had to awaken inner body sensitivities and more realistic perceptions of the self through object-directed motor activities. The expression of fantasy content in improvisations within the structure of transferences paved the way toward reintegration and acceptance of affect states and shattered interpersonal relationships.

Epilogue

ASPECTS OF DANCE
AND CHOREOGRAPHY
IN DANCE-MOVEMENT THERAPY

The entire contents of this book has been devoted to the delineation of dancelike motor behavior as a consistent and coherent treatment tool and vehicle for investigation. Drawing upon the existing structure of psychoanalytic psychotherapy, cogent concept have been extrapolated and combined with the techniques of dance-movement therapy. But no matter how great the debt to psychoanalysis may be, what is now dance-movement therapy is not a mere derivative of any verbal psychotherapy. It has its own origin in dance. Denying or diminishing this root can only be detrimental to the final efficacy of dance-movement therapy.

None of the theories and treatment tools I have developed make any sense nor can be useful if dance-movement therapists are not also firmly grounded in dance and choreography. There are certain aspects of both dance and choreography which are frequently neglected in the training of dance-movement therapists. Both classical ballet and choreography have shaped the profession. Yet, these ties are disavowed or not clearly recognized by many in the profession. Therefore these components of dance-movement therapy will be addressed in the concluding pages of this book.

Often, people who have discovered the joy of movement decide to become dance-movement therapists without appropriate dance backgrounds. They have not dealt with the basics of how to transform the motor urge and its expression into a useful, conscious form. "Useful and conscious" defines motor expression under the direction of the conscious "I" (Ego). This, quite clearly, can be as simple a move as a physical reaching out for a friend, or a complex dance. Dance-movement therapists need to include all these possibilities in their own movement repertoires.

There are basic principles involved in dance and choreography that are as structured as those in psychoanalysis. When these principles are forgotten, or have never been learned, unclear foci are presented to the client; i.e., dance-movement therapists who have not experienced the discipline and restructuring of their own body-"I" (body ego) during lengthy dance training cannot transmit the joy, safety, and order of anatomically sound motility to their clients. For instance, there are groups of dance-movement therapists who totally deny their own cultural movement heritage and origin. They are so intent on moving "organically" that they choose to move in what looks like Afro-Haitian style, or like a Hindu healing ritual rather than in the linear form, that, like it or not, is a large part of the movement expression of Western culture. Moving linearly looks balletic and therefore "inauthentic" to these visionaries without a past.

Classic dance and choreography represent the disciplined consciousness over the spectrum of motor drive and its diversified expressions in the profession of dance-movement therapy. In effect, classic dance parallels the goals of psychoanalysis when it is taught and practiced in an anatomically correct way. Psychoanalysis at its best seeks to free and promote ideal possibilities of endowment through reinforcing or creating conscious control over drives.

So does Classic Dance in its insistence on clarity of line and placement. In the purest sense of the word, it tames the motor drive under the direction of the conscious self.

Modern Dance, despite its great expressiveness, does not always aspire to such consciousness. It allows for the expression of emotion in a more direct way than Ballet. The total absence of emotion is also more clearly visible in the design and athleticism of certain dance techniques that have divorced themselves from ballet. The various modern dance idioms could be likened to flowing but shaped libidinal eruptions at one end of the spectrum, and to stern superego constructions on the other. An example of the former would be Graham's *Lamentations*, while all of Nikolai's works disavow the eloquence of private emotion. The whole midsection of modern dance presupposes knowledge of ballet as the base line from which individuation of style takes place. Such pieces as Limon's *Moore's Pavane* and Butler's *Carmina Burana* exemplify this.

Work in the area of modern dance is facilitative of dance-movement therapy but it does not include the ego ideal which is represented by ballet.

Ballet technique, applied in its most constructive aspect, produces harmony and strength. It also offers tools to contact the muscular apparatus in such a way that tension can be abreacted without undue emotional swamping, and techniques to build and reaffirm body images. Dance-movement therapists need to know ballet technique not only for their own use but in order to help clients in the manic phase to find the safety of the strict right-to-left and from-the-center movements of a simple ballet barre. Deeply regressed clients who do not know their knees or are frightened to bend them do so more readily at the barre within a structure that looks like a dance class. They also find the space above their heads and to the side more readily within the confines of *port de bras*. It is as though the clear lines of simple ballet combinations provide the external structure from which personal experimentation can take place once more. Neurotic clients also need a base line from which to distance and individuate themselves.

Again, I have found the clarity of classic ballet technique

most conducive to growth at the beginning of treatment. Despite such demonstrable growth, many dance-movement therapists do not use this approach. I am reminded of talented supervisees who categorically opposed and tried to interpret away their clients improvisations as "artificial" if these clients preferred to move in linear fashion that looked balletic. Yet to the clients their movement style felt organic. They said they wanted to attain beauty. Some others needed those arabesques and dramatic *post de bras* to indicate their great swell of feeling. Yet a third group, caught in the manic phase of their illnesses, felt safer when they could devote themselves to work at the barre.

In order to illustrate the central significance of ballet, I would like to draw attention to some of the ways in which it has an impact.

In the service of their art, ballet dancers must rebuild their body images and overcome resistances to the demands of technique, they must integrate sometimes distasteful truths about themselves, and literally make themselves into different persons than they were at the beginning of their training. The similarities to the process of dance-movement therapy are striking, as is the fact that the linear, space-cutting movements and erect, firmly held torso of ballet dancing are part and parcel of the everyday movement repertoire of the Western European tradition. It is only in the extremes of sorrow or joy that people within that tradition contract their torsos or swing their pelvises. Usually, they merely gesticulate and in every way keep their movements linear.

In addition, people strike all sorts of postures to protect themselves from a "put down," or from being dropped by someone else. A casual posture may serve autonomy by showing a potential partner that he or she is not needed. Thus they signal to the world with their bodies before they verbalize their own needs, wants, defenses, and affect states.

For the dancer, and for clients, all these components of motility must become a conscious act before a change can be affected. The classic ballet dancer in particular must overcome postural behavior patterns and internalize the technique to such an extent that an arabesque become his or her individual truthful way of pointing into the distance, a *grand jete* or leap a personal form of conquering space and gravity, and the eternally sought after "turn-out" a specific way of coming physically to terms with the continuous physical exhibition of the genital region.

The open crotch in all ballet positions not only allows for the "line" most pleasing to the balletomane but also reassures the audience that the dancer's physical prowess is not a sexual attack.

Only newborns exhibit this same innocent unconcern with their genitals, until the muscular tensions of upright posture and sphincter control force them to "turn in." It is almost as though ballet dancers sometimes hold up a physical mirror in which puritanical strivings toward freedom from sexuality is reflected. Now wonder, if this is the case, that ballet dancing is in such disrepute with that part of society that is committed to freedom for the inner drives, in particular, sexuality. Actually, turn-out could also be seen as an expression of supreme sexual self-confidence. It depends on who is turning out how.

The struggle with, for, and around sexuality takes place in practically all treatment situations within dance-movement therapy also. Like the ballet dancer who has come to terms with his or her sexuality and is therefore able to enjoy freedom from embarrassment on stage, dance-movement therapists and their clients can benefit from having worked on their turn-out. In doing so, one becomes aware of one's genital region. Incorporating one's genitals into the body image is the most complex step in development. It literally allows people to know who they are.

Turn-out in ballet, then, can be an indicator of just how comfortable and sexually self-confident one is. Conversely, it can also be used for exhibitionistic and narcissistic display.

Certain types of schizophrenics also turn out at the hips with a facility that could be a ballet dancer's envy. But such individuals usually do not know at all how to turn in. They have lost all flexibility. Ballet dancers ideally can rotate their leg from the hip socket in fulfillment of human movement potential.

The proper turnout should start in the hip socket, allowing the thighs, knees, and feet to be pointed away from each other in a horizontal line so that the performer in a correct first position facing the audience would be entirely flat. The body then must be centered above the feet between the heel and ball of the foot, with pelvis pushed forward, *derriere* tucked in, rib cage moveable but erect, and the head gracefully centered above all these carefully controlled body parts.

The ballet dancer without proper technique and a hollow back has not been able to absorb the technique entirely. He or she has perhaps learned to spin brilliantly instead, or to leap wildly in order to compensate with excessive speed and strength for the loss of personal poise. Speed and strength has been substituted where equilibrium and the harmonious, controlled interaction of all body parts was needed. Usually, such dancers do not have turn-out, and thus illustrate what happens to the body when homeostasis among the drives is not maintained. The case in point for dance-movement therapists is instructive, indeed. Where libidinal drives in the service of interpersonal relationships have not tamed aggression, the motor drive will be highly overdetermined and produce the physical ineptness, clumsiness, and even self-destructiveness seen in clients.

These brief examples demonstrate how important ballet technique is for dance-movement therapists. Another cornerstone of the profession, choreography, also does not always receive the recognition it deserves.

CHOREOGRAPHY

Just as with ballet, choreography is often undervalued in dance-movement therapy, despite the fact it is critical to the practice of the profession. Choreography, after all, is the primary form of nonverbal response dance-movement therapists offer to their clients. They are continuously confronted with the task of "choreographing" and providing movement experiences for their clients. Some clients also "choreograph" the stories of their lives. While at first these are usually improvisations, the working-through process and repetition make the improvisational story take on a choreographed quality. Others need help in giving structure to their felt experiences, or have to be presented with exercises that fit their specific needs. Dance-movement therapists respond with nonverbal interpretations that are also "choreography." Whichever way one approaches the subject, dance-movement therapists make up dances, whether consciously or unconsciously, during much of their work.

It make sense, therefore, that dance-movement therapists be familiar with choreography. The place to originate this familiarity is in dance, where choreography is built around the concepts of spatiality, rhythm, repetition, structure, and expressiveness that are also part and parcel of dance-movement therapy. Familiarity with these concepts cannot be absorbed by reading about them. They need to be experienced. An illustration of this point of view is the juxtaposition of the work of a theatrical choreographer to the process in dance-movement therapy.

Ghiselin (1955) postulated the existence of four basic characteristics that are necessary for creation: greater sensitivity to sensory stimulation, unusual capacity for awareness of relations between stimuli, predisposition to an empathy of wider range and deeper vibration than usual, and intactness of sensorimotor equipment to allow the building up of projective motor discharges for expressive functions.

This description encompasses the necessary components for interpreting both nonverbally and verbally in dance-movement therapy also, i.e., the process is the same as in an artistic production. But let us take a look at what a choreographer has to say.

I have had the opportunity to speak at length with a "prototypical" choreographer, Bruce Marks, who has allowed me to see what he perceives in himself during the act of creation.

He seems "prototypical" in that he exhibits the same concerns, joys, and agonies as others in the field.

Anxiety, or inner fragmentation, is what Bruce Marks says he feels at first when he begins to make a dance. He is the choreographer who is at this writing artistic director of Ballet West. He has given his company a number of ballets which in their storytelling classicism appear to fulfill all the magic expectations of an audience that doesn't differentiate a turn-out from a turnstile, and yet greedily clamors for the virtue and succor of "culture." On a company whose exuberant style has acquired dramatic line and lyricism under his tutelage he has set a number of ballets that he himself views as inspired by music that penetrated into his creative recesses. He also says he has a personal need to see his form of theater as a living entity that reflects the current of the times.

Pressed for detail, he speaks of "filling up the music with steps and then throwing them all out to capture the essence." Asked to become specific, he links his version of *Don Juan* to the current women's struggle for equality. He says he began to understand this link during the choreographing process when his Dona Anna, Dona Elvira, and Zerlina all were forced by the patriarchal society they lived in to use Don Juan's seduction as a catalyst for their own secret, forbidden longings. The "macho" males in their lives see them as chattels, and pawns toward their personal goals. The women are consistently portrayed as powerless to change their condition. Brutally flung about, they claim the viewers' sympathy for their enslavement.

Don Juan is Freud's classic seducer, whose inner body sensitivities have deteriorated to a point at which he needs the stimulation of a constant hunt for women to feel alive. The only one he truly loves is himself, something that Marks portrays effectively with a *Doppelgänger* who seems to spell out doom for the Don. But the Don loves himself and therefore his double. The interaction between the Don and his split-off self is one of the more erotic interplays in the ballet, and is so truthful a perception of the narcissist in action that the three beautiful and passionate *pas de deux* that the women dance with the Don pale in comparison.

The three women, pathetic and vulnerable in their eagerness to be themselves, surely conform to what Marks consciously sees them to be: symbols of the women's struggle to throw off the male yoke by whatever means at hand. But there is a possible unintended switch. The Don has split himself and re-embraced himself. Taking in his own *Doppelganger*, his own narcissistic mirror, gives him the strength to face both the women and his fate: to feel nothing. But the women are as unable to love the Don as he is unable to love them—he isn't the only narcissist aboard. As Anna and Zerlina and Elvira use him to evade their fates, so he uses them to evade his.

During their brief moments of passion in the pas de deux, Marks gives each of the women a poignant interlude of dancing herself in beauty before and with the Don. There is much reaching and many lifts, and it's all very tragic because the audience knows the perfidious seducer is about to drop the young innocent on her metaphoric head. Yet it is the women who ensnare, who eagerly look for a way out of their traps, by offering themselves as prey to a man who can no more resist seducing than they can resist being seduced.

The victims become the victimizers in a not entirely realized twist. Yet in the choreography of the scene in which the men avenge themselves and their women, Marks says exactly that with his choreography, possibly without meaning to do so. With high *ponches* the women emphasize and elongate the swords that kill their lover. In aggression, and in the grim talion principle of ancient times, men and women finally merge in a common purpose: to kill the seducer who has, after all, done no more than to concretize the longings that existed in the women before he appeared on the scene.

The split between avowed content of the ballet and the message to the audience is recognizable if one accepts the premise that gesture and technique joined in a given context mean something. In this case, the juxtaposition of manifest and unconscious content works: the tension on stage produces an electric spectacle that insists on emotional contact with the audience, who invariably respond.

In trying to answer a question for himself, Marks has answered an unintended one for the audience: the victimizer is so good at his role because he has been a victim himself. Even meeting his *Doppelgänger* head on doesn't help. He is doomed.

This somewhat lengthy account of the ballet begins to give an outline of the underlying message with which Marks seems to be struggling: how to incorporate split-off selves into one coherent whole. It is both a universal and a personal question.

The question of splits and splitting surfaces over and over again in Marks' ballets. In his *Don Quixote*, an old and a young Don confront, merge, split, and experience their universe.

In a less ambitious production Marks again tackles the question of inner splits and splitting, this time through the medium of a *Lark Ascending*. The music by Vaughn Williams sets the mood for the lyrical, at times absurd, struggles to deny gravity.

The split is there again: the lark ascends painfully, her wings are cut, she fails, and can only reach upper regions by being carried by stalwart youths who stay properly static and statuesque while she struggles.

Dichterliebe a ballet first put on with the Royal Danish Ballet, approaches the split and splitting through the medium of the lives of Heinrich Heine and Robert Shumann: their fateful, painful, melancholy relationships with their women is beautifully realized within their *Zeitgeist*. Everybody suffers deeply, joy is depicted as obscene, youth and age cannot be a progression in time and space but must confront each other with longing, split off from parts of their lives and themselves by ever-present *Weltenschmerz*.

The list goes on. Even in ballets that tell no overt story, Marks manages to set one aspect of movement against the other so that tension and splitting focus the eye of the beholder on the glittering array of kaleidoscopic motor events. Marks interprets what he sees and feels although he appears not to be aware of this. As with other choreographers, his conscious preoccupation is with movement sequences, how it will look, how it "works." He reports feeling alternately anxious and elated and grimly determined to "finish it." At the end, he feels empty and quickly looks around for another theme that will set up the same tensions and make him feel "full." Before and during his choreographic work, he immerses himself in music and hears every nuance, every phrasing acutely. His dancers' perfections and inadequacies excite him. He sees things in them that he hasn't seen before. Their potential for expressing his ideas becomes the inspiration.

In all, Ghiselin's four preconditions for creativity are met fully. Further, choreographing brings about a lessening of tension, a temporary satiety for Marks until the cycle starts again. As he sets each phrase, each combination to express his theme, he interprets, that is, the manifest content interprets, a societal theme or a linear movement problem, but it also interprets personal concerns, such as reintegration of split-off parts of the self, and taming aggression by sexuality, and above all, the split between the vision and its final execution.

That his ballets "work" seems to have as much to do with his avowed intent as with the expressed but unrecognized unconscious theme. In his creations, a fervent, sometimes grandiose, appeal is made to recognize the essential loneliness that comes with being "different" from the rest of humanity, that the very "being different" is in turn ardently to be desired in a diffused kind of way.

For artists like Marks, the externalization of the summation of life experiences appears to act as the catalyst which restores harmony to his inner economy. At the same time, his reaction to his collective world, his company of dancers and his conscious themes, seems more acutely empathic than relationships among individual and component parts of his universe. That paradox is in direct line with Greenacre's (1958) observations about "collective alternates." The increased range and deepened sensitivities of the artist in the throes of creation include heightened reactions to his own body sensations as well as to the outer world, sometimes at the expense of exclusive personal relationships. This collective love affair with the world has too often been called "the narcissism of the artist" and has been mistaken for preoccupation with technique as a distancing device. In the case of choreography, where anthropomorphizing is less prominent than in other art forms, since it deals with the human body, heightened sensory responses are of particular value.

Marks and other choreographers interpret, but also ask questions that perpetuate their personal fascination with movement in whatever style. There is no inner coming to rest for them as long as they wish to create. Their projective and explanatory actions in their artistic productions have all the components of an interpretation, in that they take pieces of a given puzzling phenomenon and rearrange the pieces until they make sense. In the same way, dance-movement therapists "interpret" nonverbally and verbally. But where the dance-movement therapist's interpretation ultimately foster resolution and harmony, the artist's and choreographer's interpretations produce this happy state only temporarily. In a way, they are their own therapists. Therefore, essential individual conflicts remain untouched and unresolved. This does not mean that art depends on neurotic conflict. It does, however, appear to need the fuel of anxiety that arises when a problem of whatever nature is unresolved; that is conflict seems necessary, but conflict is not necessarily neurotic.

To create, then, people like Marks appear to experience the following sequence of events in making a dance: recognition of emotional fragmentations within themselves; a search for a synthesizing agent, such as music or a theme; and, finally, a temporary union of all split-off elements in the finished product, the dance.

The elements that are similar in interpretation and choreography in dance-movement therapy are quite obvious. Dance-movement therapists, too, must experience inner unrest and heightened sensory awareness, they too must step outside of themselves in order to do their therapy and make their dances. There is no way a dance-movement therapist can pick up her clients' clues, nor can she respond appropriately if she does not temporarily split herself into an observing and an experiencing self in order to give total recognition to her clients' needs. The difference lies in the fact that all these inner activities are in the service of a specific other-than-self, her client, not in the service of self, nor audiences, nor even humanity. The countertransferential dilemma has been discussed. The tensions and turmoil produced by taking in another's nonverbal emanations have to reverberate within the inner world of the therapist. At best they are the stimuli which produce the unique empathic projective motor discharge which is known as dance-movement therapy. This parallels the choreographer's inner process for whom an unresolved movement theme, not a person, sparks the pre-creation fragmentation.

Quite obviously, dance-movement therapists cannot allow themselves to "love" any one client any more than a choreographer can "love" only one dancer. They need to be emotionally available to all clients and yet stay so uniquely themselves that their human kindness is diffused and given to all; as the choreographer must "give" to all the performers in the choreography, the "collective alternates" for the dance-movement therapist are all of her clients whose inner fates rest heavily against her creative receptivity.

As she choreographs for and with her clients, as the clients' fragmentation and splitting diminishes, the dance-movement therapist recaptures and recreates herself each time within her own movement repertoire. As a result it is expanded and enriched by the deep contact with another human being. The dance-movement therapist's purposeful inner fragmentation and splitting while working is, ideally, occasioned by her clients, not as is the case with some theatrical choreographers, by her own conflicts. Therefore her contribution to choregraphy must always be ephemeral, bound to the moment, and often not transmittable except to the specific client in whose life it makes sense.

Where for people like Marks a theatre dance results after

the fragmentation and splitting that is part and parcel of both processes, for dance-movement therapists the dance of concrete inner and outer reality *bourrés*, waltzers, trucks, struts, and marches into her life with her clients. And, finally, through her choreographic intervention, a reconstituted life becomes her gift to the world.

Only the two most obvious subjects, a form of dance and choreography which are vital to dance-movement therapy have been examined. It is hoped they will be road signs to the many facets of dance-movement therapists' professional lives that remain untouched, unexamined, and defended against. A collective search for a newer, more complete movement-awareness could result, an awareness that incorporates and interprets the past as the nourishing soil from which individual and collective motility can evolve.

REFERENCES

Balint, M. *The basic fault — Therapeutic aspects of regression*. London: Tavistock Publications, 1968.

Beres, O. Review of psychic trauma, *Psychoanalytic Quarterly*, (Vol. XXXVIII), 1969.

Bernstein, P. *Theory and methods in dance movement therapy*. Dubuque, Iowa: KendallHunt, 1972.

Bernstein, P. *Eight approaches to dance therapy*. Dubuque, Iowa: KendallHunt, 1979.

Bibring, E. The mechanism of depression, In *Affective Disorders*. New York: International Universities Press, 1953.

Bibring, E. Psychoanalysis and the dynamic psychoterapies. *Journal of the American Psychoanalytic Association*, (Vol. II), 1954.

Blanck, R. & Blanck, G. *Marriage and personal development*. New York: Columbia University Press, 1968.

Blanck, R. & Blanck, G. *Ego psychology I. theory and practice*. New York: Columbia University Press.

Blanck, R. & Blanck, G. *Ego psychology II Psychoanalytic developmental psychology*. New York: Columbia University Press. 1979.

Blos, P. *On adolescence*. New York: Macmillan, 1962.

Brill, A. *Freud's contribution to psychiatry*. New York: Norton, 1944.

Brody, S. Some aspects of transference resistance in prepuberty. *The Psychoanalytic Study of the Child*. (Vol. XVI) New York: International Universities Press, 1961.

Brody, S. Axelrod, S. & Moroh, M. Early phases in the development of object relations. (Vol. III), *The International Review of Psychoanalysis*, 1976.

Brody, W. M. On the dynamics of narcissim. *The Psychoanalytic Study of the Child*, (Vol. XX), New York: International Universities Press, 1965.

Brown, & Menninger, *The psychodynamics of abnormal behavior* New York: McGraw-Hill, 1949.

Cain, R. M., & Cain, N. N. A Compendium of Psychiatric Drugs. *Drug Therapy*. January 1975.

Chaiklin, H. *Marian Chace, her papers*. Columbia, Maryland: American Dance Therapy Association, 1975.

Delacato, C. H. & Dolman, G. *The Dolman-Delacato developmental profile* Philadelphia, PA: The Rehabilitation Center, 1962.

Deutsch, F. Studies in pathogenesis: Biological and psychological aspects. *Psychoanalytic Quarterly*, (Vol. II), 1933.

Deutsch, F. The Choice of Organ in Organ Neurosis. *International Journal of Psychoanalysis*, (Vol. XX), 1939.

Deutsch, F. Analytic posturology, *Psychoanalytic Quarterly*, (Vol. XXI), 1952.

Deutsch, F. Analytic synesthesiology, *International Journal of Psychoanalysis*. (Vol. XXXV), 1954.

Deutsch, F. Symbolization as a formative stage of the conversion process. *In On the mysterious leap from the mind to the body*, New York: International Universities Press, 1959.

Deutsch, H. Some forms of emotional disturbance and their relationship to schizophrenia. *Psychoanalytic Quarterly*, (Vol. XI), 1942.

Dickman, M. L., Schmidt, C. D., & Gardner, R. M. Spirometric standards for normal children and adolescents (ages five to fifteen years). *American Review of Respiratory Diseases, #104, 1971.*

Dosamantes-Alperson, E. Movement Therapy — a theoretical framework. *In Writings On Body Movement and Communication*, Columbia, MD:ADTA Monograph *#3* 1973-74.

Dosamantes-Alperson, E. Experiential Movement Psychotherapy, *American Journal of Dance Therapy* (Vol. 1), 1977.

Dosamantes-Alperson, E. The internal-external movement dimension, *American Journal of Dance Therapy*. (Vol. II), 1978.

Dosamantes-Alperson, E. The intrapsychic and interpersonal in movement psychotherapy, *Journal of Dance Therapy*. (Vol. II), 1979.

Dratman, M. & Kalish, B. Reorganization of psychic structure in autism. A study using body movement therapy. *American Journal of Dance Therapy*, 1967.

Epstein, L. & Feiner, H. *Countertransference*, Jason Aronson, New York: 1979.

Esman, A. H. The Primal Scene. *The Psychoanalytic Study of the Child*. New Haven: Yale University Press, (Vol. XXVIII), 1973.

Espenak, L. Body dynamics and dance in individual psychotherapy, *In Writings on Body Movement and Communication*, 1972 Washington, D.C.: ADTA Monograph *¿II*.

Feldenkrais, M. *Body and mature behavior*, New York: International Universities Press, 1966.

Feldman, S. Blanket interpretations. Psychoanalytic Quarterly, 1957, (Vol. XXVII).

Fenichel, O. Outline of clinical psychoanalysis. *Psychanalytic Quarterly*, 1933, (Vol. II).

Fenichel, O. Nature and classification of so-called psychosomatic phenomena. *Psychoanalytic Quarterly* (Vol. XIV) 1945.

Fenichel, O. *The psychoanalytic theory of neuroses*, New York: W. W. Nortan & Co., 1945.

Fischer, S. Body image and psychopathology. *Archives of General Psychiatry*, (Vol. X), 1964

Fliess, R. An ontogenic table *In the Psychoanalytic Reader*. New York: International Universities Press, 1948.

Freud, A. *The ego and the mechanisms of defense*. New York: International Universities Press, 1946.

Freud, A. Comments on trauma In S. Furst, (ed.) *Psychic Trauma*. New York: Basic Books, 1967.

Freud, S. *The interpretation of dreams*. (Standard Ed.) (Vol. IV & V) (Originally published, 1900) London: Hogarth Press, 1978.

Freud, S. *The psychopathology of every day life* 1901, *Standard Ed.* (Vol. VI), 1978.

Freud, S. *Fragment of an analysis of a case of hysteria*, 1905a. Standard Ed. (Vol. VII) 1978.

Freud, S. *Three essays on theory of sexuality*, 1905b. Standard Ed. (Vol. VII), 1978.

Freud, S. *Drei Abhandlungen Zur Sexual Theorie*, Sigmund Freud Studienausgabe, (Vol. V), Frankfurt a. Main: Fischer Verlag, 1975. (Originally published, 1905).

Freud, S. *On the sexual theory of children*, 1908. Standard Ed., (Vol. IX), 1978.

Freud, S. *Psychoanalytic notes on an autobiographical account of a case of paranoia.* 1911, Standard Ed., (Vol. XII), 1978.

Freud, S. *The dynamics of transference*, New York: Collier Books, MacMillan Company, 1963.(see also Standard Ed., Vol. XII) 1978. (Originally published, 1912b)

Freud, S. *Further recommendations in the technique of psychoanalysis: observations on transference love.* 1914, New York: Collier Books, MacMillan Company, 1963. (see also Standard Ed., (Vol. XII) 1978.

Freud, S. *Remembering, repeating and working through.* 1914, Standard Ed. (Vol. XII), 1978.

Freud, S. *Instincts and their vicissitudes.* 1915. (Vol. XIV). Standard Edition, (Vol. XIV) 1978.

Freud, S. *Triebe und Triebschicksal 1915.* In Sigmund Freud — Studienausgabe (Vol. III), Frankfurt a. Main: Fisher-Verlag, 1975.

Freud, S. *The unconscious.* 1915, Standard Ed. (Vol. XIV), 1978.

Freud, S. *Das Unbewusste*, 1915b., Sigmund Freud—Studienausgabe, (Vol. III), 1975.

Freud, S. *Introductory lectures on psychoanalysis, 1916* Standard Ed. (Vol. XV & XVI), 1978.

Freud, S. *Mourning and melancholia.* 1917e. Standard Ed. (Vol. XIV), 1978.

Freud, S. *Beyond the pleasure principle.* 1920, Standard Ed., (Vol. XXVIII) 1978.

Freud, S. *Jenseits des Lust Prinzips.* Sigmund Freud—Studienausgabe, (Vol. III), 1975. (Orginially published, 1920).

Freud, S. *The ego and the id.* 1923b., Standard Ed. (Vol. XIX) 1978.

Freud, S. *Splitting the ego in the process of defense*: *Inhibitions, sysptoms and anxiety.* 1926, Standard Ed., 1978.

Freud, S. *Hemmung, Sympton und Angst.* (Vol. VI). Sigmund Freud—Studienausgabe, 1975. (Originally published, 1926).

Friedman, L. The therapeutic alliance. *International Journal of Psychanalysis*, (Vol. L), 1969, #139.

Frosch, J. The psychotic character: Clinical and psychiatric consideration, *Psychiatric Quarterly*, 1949.

Gelabert, R. *Anatomy for the dancer.* New York: Danad Publishers, 1968.

Geller, J. The body, expressive movement and physical contact in psychotherapy. *In The power of human imagination.* J. Singer & K. Pape, (Ed.s) New York: Plenum Press, 1978.

Gesell, A. Y., & Amatruda, C. S., *Gesell & Amatruda's developmental diagnosis.* (H. Knoblock & B. Pasamanik, (Eds.) New York: Harper and Row, 1973.

Ghiselin, B. *The creative process.* Berkeley: University of California, Press. 1955.

Giovacchini, P. L. *Tactics and techniques in psychoanalytic psychotherapy. New York: Science House, 1972.*

Glover, E. *The technique of psychoanalysis* New York: International Universities Press, 1955.

Greenacre, P. The predisposition to anxiety. *Psychoanalytic Quarterly* (Vol. X.), 1945.

Greenacre, P. The biological economy of birth. *The Psychanalytic Study of the Child,* (Vol. I), New York: International Universities Press, 1945.

Greenacre, P. Respiratory incorporation and the phallic phase. *The psychoanalytic Study of the Child,* (Vol. VI), 1951.

Greenacre, P. Certain relationships between fetishism and faulty development of body image, *The Psychanalytic Study of the Child,* (Vol. VIII), 1953.

Greenacre, P. The Role of Transference,'' *Journal of the American Psychoanalytic Association,* (Vol. II), 1954.

Greenacre, P. The childhood of the artist: Libindinal phase development and giftedness. *The Psychoanalytic Study of the Child* (Vol. XII), 1957.

Greenacre, P. Early physical determinants in the development of a sense of identity. *Journal of the American Psychoanalytic Association, (Vol. XVI), 1958.*

Greenacre, P. The family romance of the artist. *The Psychoanalytic Study of the Child,* (Vol. XIII), 1958.

Greenacre, P. Certain technical problems in the transference relationship, *Journal of the American Psychoanalytic Association,* (Vol. VII), 1959.

Greenacre, P. Further considerations regarding fetishism. *The Psychoanalytic Study of the Child*, (Vol. XV), 1960.

Greenacre, P. Woman as artist. *Psychoanalytic Quarterly* (Vol. XXIX) 1960.

Greenacre, P. A study on the nature of inspiration: Some special considerations regarding the phallic phase, *Emotional Growth*, (Vol. I), New York: International Universities Press, 1971.

Greenacre, P. The influence of infantile trauma on genetic patterns. *In Emotional Growth*, New York: International Universities Press, 1971.

Greenberg, J. Me and Miss Chace. *In American Dance Therapy Proceedings*, 8th Annual Conference, Overland Park, Kansas, 1973.

Greenson, R. On screen defenses, screen hunger and screen identity. *Journal of the American Psychoanalytic Association (Vol. VI), 1958.*

Grinker, R. R. *Psychosomatic concepts*, New York: Jason Aronson, 1973.

Guntrip, H. *Schizoid phenomena, Object Relations and the Self.* New York: International Universities Press, 1969.

Hall, R. C. W. The Benzodiazephines. Journal of the American Psychiatric Association, (Vol. XVII), 5, 1978.

Hartmann, H. *Ego psychology and the problem of adaptation.* New York: International Universities Press, 1958.

Hartmann, H., & Kris, E. The genetic approach in psychoanalysis, *The Psychoanalytic Study of the Child*, (Vol. I), New York, International Universities Press, 1945.

Hartmann, H., Kris, E. & Loewenstein, R. M. Comments on the formation of psychic structure. *The Psychoanalytic Study of the Child*, (Vol. II), New York: International Universities Press, 1946.

Hoch, P. H. & Polatin, P. Pseudoneurotic forms of schizophrenia, *Psychiatric Quarterly*, 1949.

Hoffer, W. Mouth, hand and ego integration, *The Psychoanalytic Study of the Child.* Vol. III/IV), New York: International Universities Press, 1949.

Hoffer, W. Development of the body ego. *The Psychoanalytic Study of the Child.* (Vol. V), New York: International Universities Press, 1950.

Jacobs, T. Posture, gesture and movement in the analyst: Clues to interpretation and countertransference. *Journal of the American*

Psychoanalytic Association, (Vol. XXI), 1973.

Jacobson, E. Contribution to the metapsychology of cyclothymic depression, *In Affective disorders*, New York: International Universities Press, 1953.

Jacobson, E. The affects and their pleasure — Unpleasure qualities in relation to the psychic discharge process. *In Drive, Affect, Behavior*, R. Loewenstein, (Ed.). New York: International Universities Press, 1953.

Jacobson, E. *The self and the object world*. New York: International Universities Press, 1964.

Kernberg, O. Borderline personality organization. *Journal of the American Psychoanalytic Association* (Vol. XIX), 1967.

Kernberg, O. *Borderline conditions and pathological narcissim*, New York: Jason Aronson, 1975.

Kernberg, O. *Object Relations Theory and Clinical Psychoanalysis*. New York: Jason Aronson, 1976.

Kestenberg, J. The role of movement patterns in development. *Psychoanalytic Quarterly*, (Vol. XXXVI), 1967.

Kestenberg, J. with Berlow, J., Buelte, A., Markus, H., Robbins, E. Development of the young child expressed through bodily movement. *Journal of the American Psychoanalytic Association* (Vol. XIX), 1971.

Kestenberg, J. *Children and parents, studies in development*. New York: Jason Aronson, 1975.

Kestenberg, J. Prevention, infant therapy and the treatment of adults, *International Journal of Psychoanalytic Psychotherapy*, (Vol. VI), 1977.

Knight, R. P. *Management and psychotherapy of the borderline schizophrenic patient*: *Psychoanalytic psychiatry and psychology*, R. P. Knight & C. R. Friedman, (Ed.). New York: International Universities Press, 1957.

Kohut, H. The psychoanalytic treatment of narcissistic personality disorders, outline of a systematic approach, *The Psychoanalytic Study of Child*. New York: International Universities Press, (Vol. XXIII), 1968.

Kohut, H. *The Analysis of Self*. New York: International Universities Press, 1971.

Kohut, H. *The Restoration of the Self*. New York: International Universities Press, 1977.

Kris, E. Ego Psychology and interpretation in psychoanalytic therapy. *Psychoanalytic Quarterly*, (Vol. XX), 1951.

Kris, E. *The image of the artist, Psychoanalytic explorations in art*. New York: International Universities Press, 1952.

Kris, E. On some vicissitudes of insight in psychoanalysis, *International Journal of Psychoanalysis*, (Vol. III), 1956.

Kris, E. The recovery of childhood memories, *The Psychoanalytic Study of the Child*, (Vol. XI), New York: International Universities Press, 1956.

Krystal, H. Trauma and Affect, *The Psychoanalytic Study of the Child*. (Vol. XXXIII), New Haven: Yale University Press, 1978.

Laban, R. *The Mastery of movement*. London: MacDonald & Evans, 1969.

LeBoit, J. & Caponi, A. *Advances in the psychotherapy of the borderline patient*. New York: Jason Aronson, 1973.

Mahler, M. *On human symbiosis and the vicissitudes of individuation*. New York: International Universities Press, 1969.

Mahler, M., Pine, F., & Bergman, A. *The psychologic birth of the human infant*. New York: Basic Books, 1979.

Mittelman, B. Motility in infants, children and adults, patterning and psychodynamics, *The Psychoanalytic Study of the Child*, (Vol. IX), New York: International Universities Press, 1954.

Mittelman, B. Motor Patterns in Genital Behavior. *The Psychoanalytic Study of the Child*, (Vol. X). New York: International Universities Press, 1955.

Mittelman, B. Motility in the therapy of children and adults. *The Psychoanalytic Study of the Child*, (Vol. XII).New York: International Universities Press, 1957.

Moore, B. E., & Fine, B. D. *A glossary of psychoanalytic terms*. New York: The American Psychoanalytic Association, 1968.

Nunberg, H. *Principles of psychoanalysis*. New York: International Universities Press, 1932.

Ornitz, E. M. Disorder of perception commmon to early infantile autism and schizophrenia *Comprehensive Psychiatry*, (Vol. X). 1969.

Piaget, J. *On creativity*. Symposium at Dwight E. Eisenhower Forum, Baltimore, 1972.

Rangell, L. The psychology of poise with special elaboration on the psychic significance of the snout and perioral region. *International Journal of Psychoanalysis*, (Vol. XXXV). 1954.

Rapaport, D. *Emotions and memory*. New York: International Universities Press, 1950.

Rapaport, D., Gill, M. M., & Schaefer, R. *Diagnostic psychological testing*. Chicago: Year Book Publishing, 1945, 1953.

Reich, W. *Character analysis*. New York: Farrar, Straus & Cudahy, 1945.

Rogers, C. R. *Client centered therapy*. Boston: Houghton Mifflin Company, 1951.

Rosenfeld, H. Notes on the Psychoanalysis of the Super-ego Conflict of an Acute Schizophrenic Patient. *International Journal of Psychoanalysis,* (Vol. XXXII), 1952.

Rubenfine, D. L. Maternal stimulation, psychic structure and early object relations. *The Psychoanalytic Study of the Child*, (Vol. XVII), New York: International Universities Press, 1962.

Ruttenberg, B. A. A psychoanalytic understanding of infantile autism and its treatment. *Proceedings of Indiana University Colloquium on Infantile Autism*, Springfield, Illinois: Charles Thomas, 1971.

Rutter, M. & Schopler, E. *Autism — A reappraisal of concepts and treatment*. New York: Plenum Press, 1979.

Salzman, L. *The Obsessive Personality*. New York: Science House, 1972.

Sandel, S. Sexual issues in movement therapy with geriatric patients. *American Journal of Dance Therapy*, (Vol. III), *I*, 1979.

Sandel. S. Countertransference stress in the treatment of a schizophrenic patient. *American Journal of Dance Therapy*, 1980.

Sandler, J., & Joffe, W. G. The tendency to persistence in psychological function and development. *Bulletin of the Menninger Clinic*, (Vol. XXXI), *5*, 1967.

Sartre, P. *Being and nothingness*. New York: Philosophical Library, 1958.

Saul, L. J. Physiological systems and emotional development. *Psychoanalytic Quarterly #19*, 1950.

Schafer, R. *Aspects of internalization*. New York: International University Press, 1968.

Schafer, R. Generative empathy in the treatment situation. *Psychoanalytic Quarterly*, (Vol. XXVII), 1959.

Schilder, P. *Contributions to developmental Neuro-Psychiatry*. New York: International Universities Press, 1964.

Schilder, P. *The image and appearance of the human body*. New York: International Universities Press, 1950.

Schmais, C. Dance therapy in perspective. *Focus on Dance VII*, Washington, D.C., AAHPER, 1974.

Schmale, A. H., Jr. A genetic view of affect. *The Psychoanalytic Study of the Child*, (Vol. X), New York: International Universities Press, 1955.

Schmiedeberg, H. Kindliche Neurosen. *Zeitschrift für psychoanalytische Pädagogik*, Berlin: 1938.

Schoop, T. Philosophy and Practice. *American Dance Therapy Association Newsletter* (Vol. V), 1971.

Schur, M. The ego in anxiety. *In R. M. Loewenstein* (Ed.) *Drives, affects, behavior*. New York: International Universities Press, 1953.

Schur, M. Comments on the metapsychology of somatization. *The Psychanalytic Study of the Child*, (Vol. X). New York: International Universities Press, 1955.

Searles, H. F. Transference psychosis in the psychotherapy of chronic schizophrenia. *International Journal of Psychoanalysis*, (Vol. XXXXIV), 1968.

Searles, H. F. *Collected papers on schizophrenia and related subjects*, New York: International Universities Press, 1968.

Searles, H. H. The countertransference with the borderline patient. *In Advances in the psychotherapy of the borderline patient*. J. LeBoit & A. Capponi, (Eds.), New York: Jason Aronson, 1979.

Siegel, E. V. The resolution of breast fixation in Three Schizophrenic Teenagers. *Proceedings V*, Annual American Dance Therapy Association Conference, 1970.

Siegel, E. V. Psyche and Soma: Movement therapy. *Voices*, Special Issue, 1970.

Siegel, E. V. Developmental levels in dance-movement therapy. *Proceedings VIII*, Annual Dance Therapy Association Conference, 1973.

Siegel, E. V. Movement therapy with autistic children. *Psychoanalytic Review*, (Vol. LX), #1, 1973.

Siegel, E. V. Movement Therapy as a Psychotherapeutic tool, *Journal of the American Psychoanalytic Association*, (Vol. XXI), #2, 1973.

Siegel, E. V. Psychoanalytic thought and methodology in dance-movement therapy. *Focus on Dance VII*, AAHPER, Washington, D.C., 1974.

Siegel, E. V. Psychoanalytically oriented dance-movement therapy — A treatment approach to the whole person. *In Eight Approaches to Dance Therapy*. P. Bernstein, (Ed.), Dubuque, Iowa: Kendall/Hunt, 1979.

Siegel, E. V. & Blau, B. Breathing Together — A preliminary investigation of a motor reflex as adaptation-variability of forced vital capacity in psychotic children. *American Journal of Dance Therapy*, (Vol. II), 1978.

Spitz, R. *The first year of life*, New York: International Universities Press, 1965.

Stolorow, R. D. & Lachman, F. M. *Psychoanalysis of Developmental Arrests*, New York: International Universities Press, 1980.

Stone, L. The widening scope, *Journal of the American Psychoanalytic Association*, (Vol. II), 1954.

Wangh, M. Structural determinants of a phobia. *Journal of the American Psycholoanalytic Association*, (Vol. VII), 1959.

Whitehouse, M. The transference and dance therapy. *American Journal of Dance Therapy*, (Vol. I), 1977.

Zeigarnick, B. Über das Verhalten erledigter and unerledigter Handelungen. *Psychologische Forschung*, (Vol. IX), 1941.

Zilboorg, G. Ambulatory schizophrenia, *Psychiatry*, (Vol. IX), 1941.

INDEX